FROM ADVOCACY
TO ALLOCATION

FROM ADVOCACY TO ALLOCATION

The Evolving American
Health Care System

David Mechanic

THE FREE PRESS
A Division of Macmillan, Inc.
NEW YORK

Collier Macmillan Publishers
LONDON

The Free Press
A Division of Macmillan, Inc.
866 Third Avenue, New York, N.Y. 10022

Collier Macmillan Canada, Inc.

Printed in the United States of America.

printing number

1   2   3   4   5   6   7   8   9   10

Library of Congress Cataloging-in-Publication Data

Mechanic, David
    From advocacy to allocation.

    1. Medical care—United States—Addresses, essays,
lectures.   2. Medical policy—United States—Addresses,
essays, lectures.   I. Title.   II. Title: Health care
system.
RA395.A3M415   1986   362.1'0973   85-20431
ISBN 0-02-920830-0
ISBN 0-02-920860-2 (pbk.)

In Memory of
René Dubos,
Scientist, Scholar, Humanist:

> . . . *health and happiness cannot be absolute and permanent values, however careful the social and medical planning. Biological success in all its manifestations is a measure of fitness, and fitness requires never-ending efforts of adaptation to the total environment, which is ever changing.*

Mirage of Health, 1959

Contents

III. *The Health Professions*

IV. *The Health of Special Populations*

Preface

The American health care system is in the throes of a scientific, philosophical, and economic revolution. It is a time of ferment and uncertainty, and while we in all likelihood will maintain a pluralistic system of services, the central features of its future organization will remain in flux for some years. In the past several years I have had the opportunity to participate in a variety of health policy efforts and to write on health matters in different public forums in addition to pursuing empirical research on health and illness behavior and health care organization. The purpose of this volume is to bring together that part of my work in recent years that is directed more to policy and clinical issues than to substantive research themes in medical sociology.

While I see no disjunction between my interests in policy and clinical issues and more basic issues I research, the choice to select only a part of my work has a number of rationales. First, it allows me to assemble essays that fit together more obviously, and thus provides greater coherence as a book. But more importantly, the essays that appear here have all been published in journals and books that my social science colleagues do not typically know although they are important references for physicians, policy analysts, and policymakers in health.

Few of these essays are as they originally appeared. I have made every effort to eliminate repetition, to insure that the discussion continues to be timely, and in some cases have merged papers so as to create a different product. To provide a general context for the discussions that follow, I have prepared an introduction for the general reader that provides a brief, but hopefully clear, picture of the size, diversity, and complexity of the health care industry and its personnel.

Portions of this book have been adapted from the writings cited in the Acknowledgments and from articles published in *Health and Society: The Milbank Memorial Quarterly*. Earlier versions of some chapters were presented at conferences and appear in volumes based on these conferences.

The work reported here, and much of the research efforts on which a great deal of my thinking is based, was supported in part by the Robert Wood Johnson Foundation, the National Institute of Mental Health, the William T. Grant Foundation, and the Henry J. Kaiser Family Foundation, and I am grateful for their support. Eileen Gnecco has been extremely helpful in assisting me in bringing these essays together, putting references in common form, and helping in a variety of other details essential to completing the task in a pleasant and expeditious way.

David Mechanic
New Brunswick
October 1985

Acknowledgments

Materials from the following articles and papers, which I have written previously, have been adapted for use in this book with permission from the original publishers:

"Curing, Caring and Economics: Dilemmas of Progress," *Perspectives in Biology and Medicine* 25 (Summer 1982): 722–735, by permission of the University of Chicago Press; "Approaches to Controlling the Costs of Medical Care: Short-Range and Long-Range Alternatives," *New England Journal of Medicine* (February 1978): 249–254; "Containing Costs Through HMOs," *Colloquium: Issues in Health Care Delivery and Cost Analysis* 2 (November 1982): 1–2; "Disease, Mortality and the Promotion of Health," *Health Affairs* 1 (Summer 1982): 28–32; "Illness Behavior, Social Adaptation, and the Management of Illness," *The Journal of Nervous and Mental Disease* 165 (August 1977): 79–87, copyright 1977, Williams & Wilkins, reproduced by permission; "Public Perceptions of Medicine," *New England Journal of Medicine* 312 (January 1985): 181–183; "The Transformation of Health Providers," *Health Affairs* 3 (Spring 1984): 65–72; "A Cooperative Agenda for Medicine and Nursing" (with Linda H. Aiken), *New England Journal of Medicine* 307

(September 1982): 747–750; "Social Factors Affecting the Mental Health of the Elderly," in H. Hafner, G. Moschel, and N. Sartorius (eds.) *Mental Health in the Elderly,* by permission of Springer-Verlag, Heidelberg; "Distress and Coping in Late Adolescence," presented at the Conference on Stress Related Problems Among College Students, November 1982, by permission of The Medical Foundation, Cambridge, Mass.; and "Mental Health and Social Policy: Initiatives for the 1980's," *Health Affairs* 4 (Spring 1985): 75–88.

In each case, I am grateful to the publishers for permission to reprint these materials.

D. M.

Introduction: A Brief Anatomy of the American Health Care System

THE PURPOSE of this introduction is to present a short, overall picture of the health care system, to provide a fuller context for the chapters that follow. It is difficult to describe in brief the dimensions of an industry involving facilities, goods, and services exceeding $400 billion a year. The size, complexity, and diversity is mind-boggling; the system of care is extraordinarily dynamic; and the high stakes intimately involve hundreds of government agencies, professional groups, business interests, consumer organizations, special interest lobbies, employers and unions, public interest groups, and many others. The health industry has been growing rapidly; some estimate it will reach an expenditure level of $2 trillion and 15 per cent of the gross national product by the year 2000.

Health Expenditure Patterns and the Burden of Illness

The single major component of total health care expenditures is hospital costs, consuming 42 per cent of the total. The second-largest element is physician fees, not already included in hospital budgets, totaling slightly in excess of 19 per cent. Other major components include: nursing home care (approximately 8.5 per cent); drugs and small medical items (almost 7 per cent); dental services (6 per cent); construction of medical facilities (2.5 per cent); and administration of insurance programs (almost 4 per cent). Restricting consideration more narrowly to personal health expenditures shows that in 1983, 47 per cent of all such expenditures went for hospital care and 22 per cent for physician services. Given the size of the budget, a seemingly small 1 per cent involves expenditures of more than $4 billion.

In 1983, government at all levels accounted for 42 per cent of total health expenditures. The two largest programs, Medicare—a program for persons over 65 and a limited number of others with specific disabilities—and Medicaid—a federal-state matching program for the most impoverished part of the population—accounted for 29 per cent of personal health expenditures. Medicare alone cost $57 billion in 1983, $62½ billion in 1984, and is expected to cost $75 billion in 1985.

The pattern of health expenditures in some measure reflect the burdens of illness and risks of mortality in varying age and other social strata. The elderly and the poor are, of course, at greater risk. In examining the overall profile of mortality, four additional points ought to be considered. First, rates and causes of death vary greatly by sex and age. Women, on average, live more than seven years longer than men, and deaths among children, adolescents, and young adults are relatively low and predominantly due to accidents and self- and other inflicted violence. Second, age-adjusted death rates in the United States have been falling for major diseases with the exception of cancer. The increases in cancer are almost completely explained by smoking patterns. The large drop in age-adjusted mortality from heart disease and strokes in recent years are particularly important gains and account for a significant proportion of the advances in longevity among the American adult and elderly population. Third, while all groups in the population have benefited from downward trends in mortality, the large differentials between males and females and whites and nonwhites persist. Absolute rates have fallen, but the gaps have not significantly closed. Nonwhites and the poor remain at greater risk. Finally, while many biological, environmental, and other factors contribute to the differentials by age and sex, factors associated with behavior clearly have a major role. Cigarette smoking, accidents, excessive drinking, and failure to maintain control over blood pressure together account for massive increments in sickness and mortality.

More than two-thirds of all deaths in the United States are due to heart disease, cancer, and stroke. In excess of 7 per cent of deaths result from accidents, suicide, and homicide. Other major causes include chronic obstructive pulmonary disease (3.3 per cent), pneumonia and influenza (2.7 per cent), diabetes mellitus (1.8 per cent), chronic liver disease and cirrhosis (1.4 per cent), and atherosclerosis (1 per cent). No other single cause accounts for as much as 1 per cent of all deaths.

An alternative way of looking at the burden of sickness patterns is to examine health expenditures in relationship to varying classes of disease. Many diseases causing substantial suffering and disability, and great dependence on the medical care system, do not necessarily result in death. The 10 most costly categories of illness, as measured by expenditures on hospital care, nursing home care, professional services, and drugs, vary from circulatory disease, costing $33 billion in 1980, to endocrine, nutritional, and metabolic diseases, costing almost $8 billion. Intermediate categories, listed in order of importance were: diseases of the digestive system; mental disorders; injuries and poisoning; diseases of the respiratory system; cancer; diseases of the musculoskeletal system and connective tissues; genitourinary disorders; and diseases of the nervous system and sense organs.

The largest costs involve the elderly, who have more chronic and degenerative disorders than younger populations and require more ambulatory, hospital, surgical, and long-term care. These costs accelerate dramatically at the oldest ages and are particularly high in the final year of life. In 1977, per capita health care spending among those 65 and over was $3\frac{1}{2}$ times that of the total population, and the difference has continued to grow since then. In 1978, persons 19 and under had per capita expenditures of $286 while those 65 or older expended $2,026. Seventy per cent of all Medicare payments were on behalf of 9 per cent of the elderly involving an average payment of over $7,000. Reimbursement for the elderly was high during the last year of life, and particularly in the last 60 days before death. The 5 per cent of Medicare recipients who died in 1978 accounted for 28 per cent of program expenditures, which, on average, was $4,527 during the final year of life.

Most of the population have much of their medical expenses covered to varying degrees by health insurance. More than 90 per cent of the population have third-party insurance, most commonly profit and nonprofit insurance programs associated with the head of household's employment. The elderly are primarily covered by Medicare, and a significant proportion of the poor by Medicaid. It is estimated that in 1985 as many as 35 million people have no private or public insurance coverage. In 1982, nongovernment health insurance programs paid 29 per cent of all health care expenditures while 28 per cent were paid directly by patients. Hospital care and inpatient physician services were predominantly covered by third-party insurance, but coverage is much less comprehensive in the areas of ambulatory care, outpatient diagnostic services, drugs and appliances, preventive care, and dental and other services. Even Medicare, a program perceived as relatively comprehensive, pays only for 44 per cent of total health care costs of the elderly.[1] Out-of-pocket payments by the elderly have increased in recent years, and this population now pays a larger proportion of their total income for medical care then they did prior to the enactment of the program. Per capita out-of-pocket expenditures for the elderly are estimated to rise from $1,683 in 1985 to $2,395 by 1990. They receive, of course, much more medical care than before.

It is commonly noted that the number of poor aged has declined over time, making this age group comparable in economic status to other age categories in the population. While many elderly people have avoided poverty in large part due to social security and other public programs, a disproportionate number of aged persons live close to the poverty line and could become impoverished with cutbacks in federal programs. Moreover, the elderly group is heterogeneous. While some are affluent, many are poor. Some analysts speak of the "two faces" of aging, emphasizing that significant segments of the aged are greatly disadvantaged and face special burdens when sick. In 1981, for example, while elderly persons on average paid 13 per cent of their incomes for out-of-pocket health expenditures, the black elderly paid 23 per cent and black elderly women 27 per cent of their incomes for such out-of-pocket costs. Also, because of the inadequacy of long-term care coverage and complex eligibility criteria for Medicaid coverage, an elderly person may be required to become impoverished before the spouse can receive needed subsidy for essential long-term care. These areas continue to be important challenges for future policy formulation.

THE FOREGOING is necessarily brief since my intent is to establish a context for what follows and not to summarize this large arena. Thus, I now turn to a description of the basic components of the system: physicians, nurses, and other health care personnel; the organization of primary medical care and first contact facilities; innovative system approaches such as HMOs (health maintenance organizations); the hospital sector and related institutional facilities; tertiary care and the sophisticated teaching hospitals; and research and development in health and health care.

Health Workers

Physicians dominate the health sector although they constitute only a small minority of the many millions of health workers. At the beginning of the century there were two health workers per physician, but the present number is more like 15 to 1.[2] There are approximately one-half million physicians in the United States, a ratio of more than 1 for every 500 patients. This reflects an increase from 1.4 physicians per 1,000 patients in 1950 to 2.2 in 1985. The increasing supply reflects the substantial expansion of medical education between 1960 and 1980. In 1960–1961, American medical schools graduated somewhat less than 7,000 doctors. In recent years, they have been graduating between 16,650 and 17,400. As a consequence, we anticipate an excess future supply. The Graduate Medical Education National Advisory Committee (GMENAC), established to advise the secretary of the Department of Health and Human Services, anticipated an oversupply of 70,000 doctors by 1990 and 145,000 doctors by the year 2000.[3] The concept of oversupply is, of course, a fairly arbitrary one. In one sense, the number of doctors one needs depends on the willingness to pay for services. Much evidence supports the belief that the nation is reaching a ceiling in its financial commitment to continuing growth in the medical care sector relative to other social priorities.

Though the total supply of physicians is estimated to be in excess, some specialties are expected to be in short supply, while others are seemingly in great abundance. Areas of anticipated undersupply include general and child psychiatry, preventive medicine and emergency medicine, and physical medicine and rehabilitation. Areas expected to have large oversupply include general surgery, obstetrics-gynecology, and many of the medical and surgical subspecialties such as nephrology, rheumatology, cardiology, endocrinology, pulmonary medicine, neurosurgery, and plastic surgery. Estimates of oversupply are uncertain to some degree because many subspecialists facing inadequate specialty work loads fill in their time doing general medicine,[4] because of unanticipated changes in science and technology, and because there are alternative ways of coping with excess supply, including cutbacks in medical school enrollment, retraining doctors for needed clinical areas, expanding the boundaries of medical work, and migration of physicians to underdoctored areas. Yet when all is said, it seems evident that physician supply will be very large as compared with prior decades.

Physicians are primarily organized in relation to three major dimensions: specialty, type of group organization, and form of remuneration. All of these are in a dynamic state, and it is difficult to clearly predict future trends. A major distinction is between doctors engaged in primary care as compared with those primarily practicing specialties and subspecialties. Most typically, the primary care disciplines are defined as family practice, general internal medicine, and general pediatrics. Despite many efforts on the part of government and private foundations to encourage primary care training and practice, the trend continues toward specialty training, with a very substantial growth of medical subspecialists. On average, generalists see many more patients than specialists, charge less for each encounter, and are less likely to order complex and expensive medical procedures and laboratory tests.

Physicians have traditionally worked in office-based solo practice, and rarely in large single-speciality or multispecialty groups or other organizational settings, but the trend is clearly toward larger practice groups. In 1983, excluding physicians employed by hospitals or government, approximately half of U.S. doctors practiced by themselves, but those practicing in groups of five or more increased from approximately 17 per cent in 1975 to 23 per cent in 1983. More than three-quarters of doctors in 1983 were self-employed, varying from 87 per cent in the surgical specialties and 83 per cent in general and family practice to 68 per cent in other specialties. Older doctors are more likely to be self-employed, varying from more than four-fifths among physicians older than 56 to 61 per cent among those younger than 36. While prepaid practice is growing at a rate of 18 to 21 per cent each year, it still only serves approximately 6 to 7 per cent of the population, and thus relatively few doctors work exclusively in such settings. A much larger proportion of doctors at least have some patients covered by prepayment plans, and such coverage is becoming increasingly common. Younger physicians and women are more receptive to practice in HMOs than their counterparts.

Most doctors receive their income through fees charged for visits and specific services and procedures performed. Third-party reimbursement for doctors' fees increased from 17 per cent in 1950 to 62 per cent in 1981. In 1983, three-quarters of all doctors' patients were covered by Medicare (21 per cent), Medicaid (9 per cent), Blue Shield (23 per cent), and other private insurers (23 per cent). In 1983, doctors reported that while Medicaid covered only slightly more than half their usual fee for a follow-up office visit, Medicare paid 68 per cent and Blue Shield 77 per cent.

Even doctors working in private settings have increasingly incorporated themselves for tax and other advantages, such as limiting their financial liability. Such incorporation increased from 31 per cent of physicians in 1975 to 54 per cent in 1983. More than half of physicians working with colleagues received their remuneration in the form of a salary, while approximately a third are paid on a fee-for-service basis. Approximately 10 per cent receive a proportion of either net or gross billings. These data reinforce an important but not widely appreciated point: how practices charge patients and insurers, and how physicians within these practices are paid, are two separable matters.

The Medicare program reimburses approximately 26 per cent of office visits and almost 31 per cent of all hospital visits. Thus, Medicare, and how it pays doctors, is of crucial importance to physicians and they feel very much threatened by impending changes. Medicare is particularly important for the medical specialties accounting for 44 per cent of all visits. Average net physician income before taxes in 1983 was $106,000. It varied a great deal by specialty from a low of $68,500 for family and general practitioners to $148,000 in radiology. Incomes were lower in nonmetroplitan areas and among those who were employees as compared with those self-employed. Both the youngest and more elderly doctors earned the lowest incomes, with income highest in the 46 to 55 age group.

In summary, doctors have done rather well in the context of growing government involvement in medical care, and particularly in the context of the Medicare program. Their current status, however, is unstable due to the vigorous efforts by the government to control expenditures for medical care, reduce the federal deficit, and contain increasing costs at the state level. There is little doubt that this is an area of impending tension and acrimony, and physicians' incomes are likely to erode to some degree.

In 1980, there were about 1.3 million active registered nurses (RNs) in the United States, one for about every 145 people. The availability of RNs more than tripled since 1950, reflecting not only population changes and the increased importance of hospital care, but also the growth of technology and intensity of treatment characterizing inpatient care. Approximately two-thirds work full time and one-third part-time. Nursing is primarily based in hospitals, where two-thirds of all nurses are employed. Although most do general nursing, in recent years there have been significant increases in more specialized roles—for example, clinical nurse specialists, nurse clinicians, nurse practitioners and midwives. While very important in leadership roles in clinical settings, their number remain relatively small. In 1980, there were about 8,000 nurse clinicians, 16,000 nurse practitioners and midwives, 18,000 clinical nursing specialists, and 14,000 nurse anesthetists. Other major settings for employment of registered nurses include nursing homes, public and community health agencies, physicians' and dentists' offices, and student health services.

Nursing has become increasingly professionalized, and while in earlier eras most nurses obtained three-year diploma degrees and two- and three-year associate degrees, most nurses are now educated in colleges and universities. While in 1980 only a third of all practicing nurses had baccalaureate degrees, a major goal of nursing is to eventually require the baccalaureate for entry into practice. Many nurses are also going on for graduate degrees as well.

Unlike physicians, nurses are primarily employees, paid through hospitals and other institutional or agency settings. Nursing salaries have been traditionally low, often on a par with secretaries and other female workers, but lower than teachers and social workers. While salaries vary to some extent depending on supply and demand for nurses and the ability of nurses to organize and conduct effective collective bargaining, nursing salaries are constrained both by the large potential supply and the cost pressures on hospital budgets. Nurses, despite their crucial importance to the sophisticated care of the critically ill, earn between one-fifth and one-sixth of physicians' incomes. Of even greater import is the absence of income-graded career structures in clinical nursing, allowing little income differentiation between the young starting nurse and the more experienced nurse. While various aspects of the economics of nursing are hotly debated, it seems clear that many nurses leave nursing or reduce their level of participation because of relatively low pay. This, in combination with responsibility for important on-the-spot clinical judgments but with little clinical autonomy, and gruelingly hard work, makes nursing less attractive to many talented and ambitious people who see better alternative career prospects, or to older nurses who may drop out as they find the physical and psychological demands too heavy for the rewards they receive.

While nursing care provided by RNs are the key to high-quality patient care in hospitals, their efforts are supported by large numbers of licensed practical nurses and nursing aides and orderlies. In 1978, half a million licensed practical nurses and 1.1 million aides and orderlies supplemented registered nursing. Hospitals in 1978 also employed 240,000 laboratory personnel, 104,000 workers in radiological services, 80,000 in medical records, 52,000 respiratory therapy workers, and innumerable others carrying out such varied functions as billing, speech therapy, physical therapy, dietary services, etc. Even a cursory examination of the range of hospital employees conveys the enormous complexity of hospitals, their technologies, and their managerial responsibilities and challenges. Dentistry constitutes a separate system to a considerable extent, but it is worth noting that by 1980 we had in excess of 144,000 dentists and 230,000 dental hygienists, assistants, and laboratory technicians.

The Hospital

With the emergence of intensive and sophisticated surgical and critical care technologies, the hospital has become the central focal point of the medical care system. Not only does the hospital provide the context, technology, and specialized personnel for a broad array of medical applications, it also often serves as the core element in a system that includes ordinary primary care services, specialized ambulatory clinics, home care programs, affiliated nursing homes, rehabilitation programs, and a wide array of other services. In 1983, there were 6,888 hospitals in the United States, accounting for

1,350,000 beds, almost 39 million hospital admissions, and more than 270 million outpatient visits. While the numbers of hospitals has not changed much in several decades, and the number of beds has been reduced by several hundred thousand in the past 20 years, the hospital's sophisticated capacities have accelerated rapidly, making the institutions of the 1950s and those of the present vastly different. As previously noted, two-fifths of all medical care expenditures—approximately $160 billion in 1984—are for hospital services.

The most typical component of the hospital system is the 5,789 community hospitals, acute short-stay institutions accounting for almost 900,000 beds in 1983, somewhat in excess of four beds per 1,000 persons in the population. Most of these hospitals have between 50 and 200 beds, although 613 hospitals have in excess of 400 beds. Because of both technology and the need for economies of scale, the average size of community hospitals has been growing, increasing from an average of 153 beds in 1972 to 176 beds in 1983. Other hospitals, in 1983, included 342 federal hospitals and 703 special hospitals, such as long-term care institutions, psychiatric hospitals, chronic disease hospitals, and hospitals for respiratory diseases, alcoholism, mental retardation, and so on.

In 1983, on any given day, there were 750,000 patients in community hospitals, an occupancy rate of 73.5 per cent, staying an average of 7.6 days. With aggressive cost-containment efforts, hospital admissions and length of stay have been falling, with occupany rates dropping to 68 per cent by mid-1984. The average cost per day of providing inpatient care in 1982 was $369, of which more than half went for personnel other then interns, residents, and other trainees. Intensive and coronary care beds are about 6 per cent of all beds, but cost $2\frac{1}{2}$ times the regular bed charge. In 1982, the average cost for an intensive care bed was $408 a day in contrast to $167 for a regular bed.[5] Averages, of course, hide extraordinary variations among institutions by geographic area, size, patient mix, type of sponsorship and control, as well as many other factors.

Although data beyond 1983 are limited, admissions to voluntary hospitals declined from 1983 to 1984 from more than 36 million to approximately 35 million, a drop of almost 4 per cent. Average length of stay also decreased from 7 to 6.7 days among the nonelderly population and from 9.6 days to 7.4 days among patients covered by Medicare. Despite a reduction in hospital beds, occupancy rates declined to about two-thirds of capacity, a rate sufficiently low to induce great alarm among hospital administrators. While it is too early to fully assess this trend, or to provide an adequate empirically substantiated explanation, one major change has been a shift in surgical procedures from the hospital to ambulatory surgi-centers. A major strategy of for-profit industries and major suppliers is to put emphasis on surgical procedures that can be used in ambulatory settings, thereby avoiding the necessity of hospitalization. American Hospital Supply, for example, has developed lasers and a special new eye lens that allows cataract removal on an outpatient basis. Such transfer of technologies from the hospital, involving several days of inpatient care, to outpatient settings has dramatic cost implications since cataract surgery is one of the most commonly used surgical procedures with the elderly population.

There is much speculation about the recent drop in hospital admissions and length of stay. While some attribute the effect to the initiation of a diagnostic-related group (DRG) methodology under the Medicare program, the drop preceded its implementation and is unlikely to explain the change. It is more likely that impending cost constraints in general, anticipation of DRGs, the tougher activities of peer review organizations that assess the necessity for hospital admission, and the overall influence of increased cost-consciousness have all contributed to a more thorough scrutiny of the necessity for inpatient care. Moreover, the profitability of ambulatory surgery and other technical procedures for health companies and physicians must be taken into account. Medicare data for the years 1977–1982 show astronomical increases in the numbers of services and procedures performed, ranging from routine urinalysis, blood sugar tests, and examination of the feces for occult blood to EKGs and their interpretation. Understanding changes in hospital patterns requires examining the changing mix between services provided in hospitals and in ambulatory settings.

Hospitals have traditionally been owned and operated by a variety of governmental, community nonprofit, religious, and proprietary organizations. The dominant form has been the voluntary not-for-profit hospital, organized under the auspices of community groups, religious orders, and a variety of other groups—for example, unions and industrial organizations, cooperatives, and organizations such as the Shriners. A small segment of the industry has been owned by individuals, partnerships, and investors seeking profits and there has been a long and continuing debate about the contributions and costs of having a proprietary sector in health care. This debate has very much accelerated in recent years with the aggressive entry of large multihospital corporations and other large investor-owned facilities. Contentions vary greatly: some argue that these developments bring new services to populations presently lacking them and force greater efficiencies in hospitals specifically and the health industry more generally; others contend that these profit-oriented ventures "cream" the profitable illnesses and patients, leaving higher risk patients and those with nonprofitable conditions to the public sector. They also argue that the powerful profit motives of medical care corporations, and their potential influences over practitioners, will significantly alter the way medicine is practiced and decisions are made in the future.[6]

The debate will continue. One fact, however, is clear: profit corporations in health care operations are growing at a rapid rate. As of 1982, approximately 10 per cent of hospitals were owned and 4 per cent were managed by profit chains; another 5 per cent were independently owned proprietaries.[7] These numbers are less impressive than the fact that the number of hospitals owned or managed by for-profit chains doubled between 1976 and 1982 and such corporations are aggressively acquiring existing hospitals, constructing new ones, and taking over small proprietary enterprises. In 1985, Hospital Corporation of America (HCA), the largest such chain, owned or managed 431 hospitals accounting for in excess of 60,000 beds. In 1983, HCA had operating revenue of almost $4 billion and earnings per share that have increased for 15 straight years, yielding a compound annual earnings per share growth rate of 25 per cent.[8] In 1984, HCA had net income of almost $300 million on net revenue of $3.5 billion and was devoting considerable resources to acquire and build more hospitals. As of 1983, Humana Corporation averaged growth in earnings per share of 41 per cent, and American Medical International 26 per cent. In sum, as Richard Rosett has put it, whether or not these corporations "are doing good, they are certainly doing well."[9]

In addition to the growth of chains of institutions, known as horizontal integration, there are increasing efforts by the health industries to increase their span of involvement over the entire array of health services, facilitating greater control over their markets, sources of supply of patients and products, and interorganizational relationships. In April 1985, a merger was proposed between HCA and

American Hospital Supply Corporation, the largest source of medical supplies, which makes and distributes 130,000 products. The combined revenues of these companies in 1984 totaled $7.6 billion.* HCA as of 1985 owned 17 per cent of shares in Beverly Enterprises, the largest nursing home chain, and it is anticipated that the continuation of vertical integration will proceed by acquiring companies manufacturing drugs, medical technologies, and ambulatory services and products. Humana, the third largest hospital chain, is marketing health insurance—Humana Care Plus—which provides a patient population for the facilities they own. While mergers and integration of programs and facilities are a response to the changing and more constrained economic environment, and an aggressive effort to take advantage of new opportunities, it also characterizes the new and influential constellation of forces in the health care arena.

It is difficult to forecast future developments, but generally two rather different scenarios are predicted for the future. Some anticipate accelerated development of profit-oriented ventures with corporate chains taking over many more hospitals and other types of health care facilities, integrating them into systems, and setting the tone for the medical care marketplace overall. It is suggested that in a decade or two, six or seven large corporations will dominate hospitals and much of the industry, and physicians significantly will be proletariatized. Alternatively, others believe that such firms will control a stable segment of the market, but not dominate it, preferring to invest in selected areas where opportunities are more promising of profits in an environment increasingly characterized by cost-consciousness and cost-regulation.

Ambulatory Medical Care

Ambulatory medical care is carried out in a variety of settings including doctors' offices, clinics, hospital outpatient departments, single-speciality and multispecialty group practices, prepaid group practices, independent practice organizations, health centers, and emergency rooms. A variety of factors affect where people come for care including the availability and accessibility of providers, ability

*The proposed merger between HCA and the American Hospital Supply Corporation failed when Baxter Travenol, a hospital supply company, offered a higher price for AHSC stock. Pressures from stockholders resulted in acceptance of the Baxter offer.

to pay and insurance status, attitudes and knowledge, and personal taste. There is broad agreement that it is desirable that patients have a primary care service that monitors their continuing needs for care, provides basic services, and makes referrals when necessary. This service should provide most basic preventive and acute care, coordinate whatever specialty care is used, and serve as patients' ombudsmen, helping them negotiate the complexities of the system.

Only some ambulatory care settings provide primary care in the sense described. Many are simply points of first contact, making an initial assessment of the patient's complaint and referring the patient as needed. While the patient may or may not come back to this setting, the physicians involved do not necessarily view themselves as the patient's personal physician or has having responsibility for continuity of care. Other services of first contact, such as outpatient departments in hospitals or emergency rooms, typically provide episodic care with little continuity and with little assumption of the role of personal physician for coordinating the patients' medical needs. Patients using such sources of care may see different doctors each time or may be treated for a single condition with little attention to other problems and needs they may have. While such care may not be optimal, even patients having alternatives sometimes choose to seek care from these settings, suggesting the variability and complexity of patient preferences.

Some settings are organized to provide primary medical care services more consistent with the definition stated earlier. Among physicians, the specialties of family practice and general internal medicine espouse such philosophies, and for children and adolescents, many pediatricians typically take similar responsibilities. Among organized practices, those emphasizing a "gatekeeper" role for the physician of first contact, such as prepaid group practice and independent practice organizations, often have highly developed approaches to primary care, although much variation exists in how broadly the physician of first contact construes his or her responsibilities and the degree of continuity of care with a physician who knows the patient. In many large health maintenance organizations, for example, continuity of care may be more developed in theory than reality, and patients with a need for acute care may commonly see an "urgent care" physician other than their designated primary care doctor.

The National Ambulatory Medical Care Survey (NAMCS)[10] provides data on encounters with office-based physicians. Office-based general and family practitioners account for about one-third of all visits and internal medicine and pediatrics for approximately another 25 per cent. Specialists also provide much general care in addition to care in their special domains. Using estimates from NAMCS, the average patient made 2.6 office visits in 1981, varying from 2.1 visits among those under 15 years to 4.3 visits for those 65 and over. Women made more visits than men. Somewhat more than a third of the visits were for acute problems, 28 per cent for routine chronic problems, and about 18 per cent for nonillness care. Other major reasons were for flare-ups of chronic conditions (9 per cent) and postsurgical or postinjury care (9 per cent). The vast majority of patients seen were previous patients (86 per cent) with old problems (64 per cent). Twenty diagnoses accounted for two-fifths of all care. The five most common were: essential hypertension (4.9 per cent); normal pregnancy (4.3 per cent); health supervision of an infant or child (3.2 per cent); acute upper respiratory infection (2.5 per cent); and general medical exam (2.4 per cent). Other frequent diagnoses included ear infections and diabetes mellitus. The above data are based on diary studies completed by office-based doctors. An alternative approach is to survey the population to assess their access to and use of health services. Data collected in 1982 indicate that 90 per cent of those surveyed report a usual source of care, and 80 per cent saw a physican at least once in the previous 12 months.[11]

The data described earlier relate to visits in doctors' offices, but patients see doctors in other contexts as well. In 1981, 69 per cent of all visits with doctors were in their offices, 13 per cent were in hospital outpatient departments, and 12 per cent of consultations were over the phone. Using a broader definition of visits, including these three types, the average number for the population was 4.6, and was highest among children under six, the elderly, and women.[12] The most common complaints seen, of course, vary by specialty.[13] Among family practitioners, for example, the five most frequent reasons for a visit (examination, acute upper respiratory infection, hypertension, prenatal care, and diabetes mellitus) accounted for almost one-fifth of all visits. The five most common complaints seen by a gastroenterologist accounting for a comparable proportion of visits included chronic enteritis and ulcerative colitis, functional disorders of the intestines, diseases of the esophagus, cirrhosis of the liver, and ulcer of the duodenum.

Health Maintenance Organizations

Health maintenance organizations (HMOs) still serve only a small minority of the population, but they are growing rapidly and are commonly seen as a prevalent model for the future. A major advantage to consumers is its prepayment feature and the availability of comprehensive services with little or no out-of-pocket costs. Government advocates see the HMO as an attractive model because of its implicit incentives to maintain a low rate of hospital admissions. At last count there were almost 17 million enrollees in HMOs, and enrollments have been growing yearly at a hefty 18 to 21 per cent. Between June 1983 and June 1984, HMO membership increased by 21.2 per cent. In 1984, there were 28 plans with 100,000 or more subscribers, as compared with 19 plans in 1982.[14] As of June 1984, these plans accounted for 58 per cent of total HMO enrollment. Average (mean) plan size, in contrast, was just below 50,000 members as of 1985. The majority of plans are relatively small in membership but are expected to grow substantially in future years. HMOs develop more rapidly in large urban settings characterized by mobility of population, and have become particularly well established in California and the Northwest and in various Northcentral states, particularly Minnesota and Wisconsin.

HMOs come in a great variety of forms, making the term itself somewhat misleading. Though they all have prepayment in common, almost every other dimension varies from one to another. While traditional established plans, such as Kaiser-Permanente and the Health Insurance Plan (HIP) of New York, were organized around group practice—hence the rubric prepaid group practice—many independent practice associations have doctors providing services to enrollees in their private offices. Even among traditional prepaid practices, some, Kaiser-Permanente for example, build, own, and operate their own hospitals, while others, such as HIP, use community hospitals. Physicians in prepaid groups are organized as staff employees in some HMOs, while in others they constitute self-governing groups that contract with the health care plan. Some large prepaid groups almost exclusively serve enrollees, while others mix prepaid and fee-for-service patients. While many HMOs are nonprofit organizations, for-profit HMOs are now a growth industry. In short, knowing that an organization is an HMO conveys relatively little about its philosophy, structure, functioning, or quality.

Hospital Use

Rates of admission to hospitals vary enormously from one area to another and cannot be explained by the populations served or patterns of need, illness, or disability. Criteria for hospital admission and length of stay are commonly ambiguous and depend as much on the experience and judgment of the individual physician and local practices as they do on established professional norms. Tougher criteria for hospital admission, earlier ambulation following surgery, reduced length of stay, and performance of many types of surgery on an outpatient basis, all attest to the ability to substantially change customary practice with few negative effects and often positive medical as well as economic benefits.

A major use of hospitals is for surgical procedures; in 1979, almost 30 million procedures were performed on almost 19 million patients in short-stay hospitals.[15] The most common surgical procedures, each performed at least half a million times were: episiotomy, diagnostic dilatation and curettage of the uterus, endoscopy of the urinary system, bilateral destruction or occlusion of the fallopian tubes, cesarean section, tonsillectomy, and repair of inguinal hernia. The average length of stay of patients receiving procedures was 7.2 days in 1979, with the hospital stay varying by type and number of procedures.

Surgical rates vary by age and sex, with the highest rates among the elderly and women. Young males under 15 have more surgery because of accidents and injuries, but in the age group 15 to 44, the rate among females is approximately four times that among men. Even if obstetrical procedures are excluded, the rate among women far exceeds that among men, largely due to procedures related to the female reproductive system. In the age group 45 to 64, the female rate is still higher but much closer to the male rate (1,746 as compared with 1,509 per 10,000 population). In the age group over 65, male rates are considerably higher (3,056 versus 2,256 per 10,000 population). These differences reflect the higher prevalence of procedures for men relating to the respiratory and cardiovascular systems. Older men also have more procedures than women affecting the urinary system. Procedures related to obstetrics or the reproductive system account for two-fifths of all female procedures, while male procedures predominate in the areas of the digestive system, the musculoskeletal system, and the urinary system.

Diagnostic procedures performed on inpatients are frequently performed on outpatients as well, and thus understate the total prevalence. In 1979, 2.4 million biopsies and endoscopies were performed on inpatients. Other common procedures were radioisotope scans, arteriography, myelograms, and intravenous pyelograms. In 1979, there were almost 200,000 CAT (computerized axial tomography) scans on inpatients; the frequency of such scans seem to be increasing rapidly as this type of radiography becomes a fairly conventional hospital technology. Such units are also increasingly available in offices of large medical practices.

Wennberg and Gittelsohn[16] have documented large variations in available resources and the amount of care given from one locality to another. In one analysis of variations among 13 hospital service areas in Vermont, for example, they documented extraordinary differences by area in hospital discharges (from 122 per 1,000 to 197), surgical procedures (from 36 to 69 per 1,000 population), available hospital beds per 10,000 persons (34 to 59), hospital personnel per 10,000 people (68 to 120), and so on. Their work suggests the importance of establishing clear norms within the medical profession describing reasonable ranges for resource need, hospital admission, and surgical intervention. Geographic, economic, and social differences would lead us to expect some variability, and uncertainty in medical practice is a reality we cannot wish away, but it is difficult to believe that with careful planning, education, and peer review we cannot more effectively limit the enormous range of these discrepancies. Some areas may have too few resources and fail to provide all the care needed, but most knowledgeable observers believe that these variations in large part reflect excess hospital beds, an overabundance of physicians and surgeons in particular areas, and incentives that encourage additional procedures and interventions at the margins.

Long-Term Care

The long-term care industry and nursing homes as its dominant institution are not new, but they grew rapidly in response to the infusion of funds that followed the implementation of Medicaid in 1966. In 1960, only $500 million a year was expended in nursing home care, approximately 2 per cent of total personal expenditures for health care. In 1983, the comparable numbers were more than 9 per cent and approximately $29 billion. As of 1980, there were an estimated 23,000 facilities fitting the description of a nursing home, with approximately 1.5 million beds. As of the same year, the Government Accounting Office estimated the availability of 1,373,300 licensed nursing home beds.[17] Nursing homes are relatively small; the average in 1980 was 66 beds. Medicare only covers short-term skilled nursing and rehabilitative care and, in 1979, contributed only 3 per cent of nursing home expenditures. Medicaid, in contrast, has substantially become the nation's long-term care financing mechanism, contributing 45 per cent of all nursing home expenditures in 1979. In 1977, Medicaid supported to varying degrees between 48 and 75 per cent of all nursing home patients. Slightly less than half of all nursing home expenditures are privately financed.

The vast majority of nursing homes in the United States are proprietary institutions; of the 18,900 facilities included in the National Nursing Home Survey of 1977,[18] 14,500 were owned by private groups. These vary from the small "mom and pop" type operations, which are believed to constitute about 40 per cent of the total, to large corporate chains. For example, Beverly Enterprises as of 1985 owned 908 nursing homes. In 1984 Beverly earned almost $47 million on revenues of $1.4 billion.

The vast majority of patients in nursing homes are old and infirm and require assistance in many of the activities of daily living. In 1977, almost 600,000 patients had difficulties with incontinence, more than 400,000 required assistance in eating, and a majority required assistance in walking, in using the toilet, in dressing, and in bathing. Patients most commonly suffer from diseases of the circulatory system and mental disorders and senility. In 1977, only 4,200 facilities provided registered nurses on all shifts, and an additional 2,400 had registered nurses on duty for two shifts. Many institutions depend heavily or even exclusively on licensed practical nurses or even nurses' aides. While most institutions have an arrangement with a person who fills the title "medical director," most physicians spend little or no time in these institutions and the quality of care depends almost exclusively on the competence level and quality of the nurses who work there.

As they get older, the elderly are at much greater risk of institutionalization. The aging of the American population, and particularly the large increases in the population over age 85, suggests that we will need many more nursing home beds or must develop viable home care and other community alternatives if we are to escape significant expansions of the existing nursing home industry. Important alternatives are to convert unused or excess hospital bed capacity for long-term care; to develop grades of supervised housing in the community with adequate nursing, medical, and social service backup; and to develop and expand programs to enhance social functioning among the aged, to assist families who assume much of the ongoing care, and to remedy the social isolation of many frail elderly people. In coming years, long-term care considerations will increasingly dominate the nation's health and social services agenda.

Systems Within Systems: Federal Health Services

In addition to financing much of the public's health care, the federal government also owns, operates, or provides for relatively complete systems of services for veterans (Veteran's Administration), armed forces personnel and their dependents (Department of Defense), and American Indians (Bureau of Indian Affairs). This is not the context for any detailed discussion of these systems, but it is useful to provide some sense of their magnitude and scope.

The VA medical care system was originally developed to aid veterans with service-connected problems and disabilities, but over time, the system expanded to serve many others. In 1981, 84 per cent of VA patients were treated for health problems unrelated to military service. As of 1983, the VA operated 172 hospitals, 226 outpatient clinics, and 99 nursing home units.[19] Its department of medicine and surgery alone employed 194,000 persons. During 1981, the VA served approximately 1.3 million inpatients, 42,000 nursing home patients, and provided almost 18 million outpatient visits. Its expenditures for 1983 were almost $8 billion, and large future increases are anticipated with the aging of our veteran population. The VA has developed a blueprint for meeting anticipated needs that would require increases of personnel by 70 to 150 per cent by the year 2000. With growing concern about government health budgets, various proposals have been made to integrate the VA system into our larger medical care system, to cut back on the scope of services offered to veterans with nonmilitary-related health problems, and to screen patients more carefully on the basis of their ability to pay their own medical care expenses. While some cutbacks and changes in service patterns are possible, veterans' groups constitute a powerful and effective lobby that have successfully thwarted such initiatives in the past.

The Department of Defense (DOD), in contrast, directly serves existing military personnel and provides for core dependents under the Civilian Health and Medical Program of the Uniformed Services (CHAMPUS), which authorizes care in non-DOD facilities when necessary services are not easily available in DOD installations. CHAMPUS operates like an insurance program with cost-sharing between the DOD and the recipient. It is estimated that the DOD provides service for 9 million persons, including both active and retired military personnel, their dependents, and survivors. In 1983, the DOD operated 161 hospitals and 310 clinics in the United States and abroad. Its medical care expenditures in 1982 were almost $7 billion, including the estimated provision of almost 900,000 hospital admissions and more than 51 million outpatient visits. The Indian Health Service, a considerably smaller program, operates 47 hospitals and 172 clinics for American Indians and Alaska natives.

The Health Care Research Establishment, American Medical Schools, and the Teaching Hospital

The federal health research establishment, concentrated in the National Institutes of Health (NIH), and intimately linked with research efforts in medical schools, teaching hospitals, and universities is one of the most admired achievements of our national government. It has received sustained support from the public and the Congress, and the NIH alone has a budget in excess of $5 billion. In addition, extensive research and related efforts are supported by the Alcohol, Drug Abuse and Mental Health Administration (ADAMHA), consisting of three institutes relating to mental health, alcoholism, and drug abuse.

The NIH is organized around 12 bureaus and institutes that range widely over categorical disease areas and health concerns. The largest institutes include the National Cancer Institute, the National Heart, Lung and Blood Institute, and the National Institute of Arthritis, Diabetes and Digestive and Kidney Disease. The other institutes vary from broad general areas—such as aging, child health and development, the environmental health sciences, and general medical sciences—to more specific concerns—such as allergy, and infectious disease and dental research. Much of the basic and applied medical research in universities and medical schools is supported through the NIH extramural research program, involving a process where investigators submit requests for grants that are then evaluated by committees of peers rated on the basis of scientific merit. Proposals receiving the best priority scores are funded consistent with the availability of funds. In 1982, NIH contributed 20 per cent of all national basic research support, 37 per cent of all such federal support, and 48 per cent of all basic research support to universities and colleges.[20] The NIH also operates a vigorous intramural research program and supports research training and other research-related programs. More than half of all NIH funding goes to medical schools, and most of that goes to a relatively small group of elite institutions. In 1982, the top 20 medical schools accounted for half of all NIH support, and the top 10 for about one-third of all NIH support.

There are 127 medical schools in the United States. These schools have affiliation agreements with approximately 1,000 hospitals, but 100 of these hospitals account for about half of all residents trained. Thus, there are very major differences among institutions designated as teaching hospitals. Sixty-one hospitals share common ownership with medical schools, and for most purposes can be viewed as components of the same institution. Medical schools and major teaching hospitals also play an important part in the education of nurses, dentists, pharmacists, and other health professionals, and are important centers for research and training. The total effort is often given the title of Health Sciences Center.

Medical schools and teaching hospitals expanded rapidly in recent decades with the infusion of large sums of research support from the NIH. Seen as on the cutting edge of medical science, new technology, sophisticated patient care, and an investigatory mode, this perspective encouraged increasing specialization and subspecialization and a high dependence on the clinical laboratory and newly developed diagnostic procedures. Because of their sophistication, many teaching hospitals attracted a sicker and more complex mix of patients, and the process of training students and residents in these institutions contribute to a more expensive pattern of care than that found in the typical nonteaching community hospital.

As efforts are made to constrain expenditures for hospital care through rate regulation, diagnosis-related group methodologies, and other devices, there is growing concern among medical educators that new forms of reimbursement will not adequately pay teaching hospitals for their complex and sicker mix of cases, for their crucial role in training future generations of medical students, residents, and other health professionals, for the magnitude of uncompensated care they provide for the indigent without insurance, and for the intangible costs associated with maintaining sophisticated research operations. Our key teaching hospitals are a major national asset, and the way of reimbursing them fairly for their varied service, educational, and research functions are difficult issues. Balancing the preservation of their unique role in our health care system on the one hand, but also avoiding unnecessary costs on the other, will probably only evolve through a process of trial and error. We probably require a much more sophisticated classification of teaching hospitals, since many have only a modest teaching and research role.

There are those who believe that the technical orientation of our teaching hospitals, and their emphasis on the more rare and complex diseases, distort medical education and the health care system. They argue that the teaching hospital should play a larger and more central role in preventive medicine and primary medical care, assisting in better preparing young health professionals for the typical problems they are likely to confront in practice,[21] and teaching practice strategies that prevent illness and disability and promote functioning among the chronically ill. While these are all goals of much importance to our medical care system, it is unlikely that teaching hospitals will take a primary role in meeting these challenges; nor is it obvious that they should do so. Teaching hospitals serve a unique function in caring for the very sick, as well as expanding our knowledge of how to do so more effectively.

Medical care in America requires a better balance between prevention and treatment, promotion of function and cure, and educational as compared to technical approaches to care. We should not, however, confuse the need for a more sober balance with denigration of the search for more sophisticated treatments and better understanding of disease processes. It is the combined agenda of balance and scientific sophistication that offers us the greatest potential for a system of effective medical care for the future.

References

1. Aiken L, Bays K. The Medicare debate—round one. N Engl J Med. 1984; 311:1196–1200.
2. Ginzberg E. Allied health resources. In: Mechanic D, ed. Handbook of health, health care, and the health professions. New York: Free Press, 1983:479–494.
3. U.S. Department of Health, Education and Welfare. GMENAC staff papers: supply and distribution of physicians and physician extenders. Washington, D.C.: Government Printing Office, 1978.
4. Aiken L, et al. The contribution of specialists to the delivery of primary care. N Engl J Med. 1979; 300:1363–1370.
5. Congress of the United States, Office of Technology. News release, Nov. 29, 1984.
6. Starr P. The social transformation of American medicine. New York: Basic Books, 1982.
7. Gray B, ed. The new health care for profit: doctors and hospitals in a competitive environment. Washington, D.C.: National Academy Press, 1983:2.
8. Wohl S. The medical industrial complex. New York: Harmony Books, 1984.
9. Rosett R. Doing well by doing good: investor-owned hospitals. University of Chicago: Michael Davis Lecture, Center for Health Administration Studies, Graduate School of Business, 1984:3.
10. National Center for Health Statistics. Patients' reasons for visiting physicians: national ambulatory medical care survey, U.S. 1977–78. Hyattsville, Md.: National Center for Health Statistics, 1981. (DHHS publication no. 82–1717, Series 13, No. 56.)
11. Robert Wood Johnson Foundation. Special report, update on access to health care for the American people. Princeton, N.J.: Robert Wood Johnson Foundation, 1983, No. 1.
12. National Center for Health Statistics. Health—United States, 1983. Hyattsville, Md.: National Center for Health Statistics, 1983. (DHHS publication no. [PHS] 84–1232:137.)
13. Robert Wood Johnson Foundation. Special report, medical practice in the United States. Princeton, N.J.: Robert Wood Johnson Foundation, 1981.
14. National Industry Council for HMO Development. The health maintenance organization industry ten-year report, 1973–1983.
15. National Center for Health Statistics. Surgical and nonsurgical procedures in short-stay hospitals: United States, 1979. Hyattsville, Md.:

National Center for Health Statistics, 1983. (DHHS publication no. [PHS] 83–1731, Series 13, No. 70:3.)

16. Wennberg J, Gittlesohn A. Small area variations in health care delivery. Science. 1973; 182:1102–1108.

17. U.S. General Accounting Office. Constraining national health care expenditures: achieving quality care at an affordable cost. Sept. 30, 1985.

18. National Center for Health Statistics. The national nursing home survey: 1977 summary for the United States. Hyattsville, Md.: National Center for Health Statistics, 1979. (DHEW publication no. [PHS] 79–1794, Series 13, No. 43.)

19. Veteran's Administration. Caring for the older veteran. Washington, D.C.: Government Printing Office, 1984.

20. National Institutes of Health. NIH data book. Bethesda, Md.: Office of Planning and Evaluation and the Division of Research Grants, June 1984.

21. Lewis J, Sheps, C. The sick citadel: the American academic medical center and the public interest. Cambridge, Mass.: Oelgeschlager, Gunn and Hain, 1983.

Bibliographic Note

For the purposes of this introduction it is superfluous to document each of the figures or trends noted. Only occasional references are given. Much of the data in the chapter can be found in the following general data sources: National Center for Health Statistics, *Health—United States, 1983,* Washington, D.C.: U.S. Government Printing Office, DHHS Pub. No. (PHS) 84–1232, Dec. 1983; *Health—United States, 1984,* Washington, D.C.: U.S. Government Printing Office, DHHS Publ. No. (PHS) 85–1232, Dec. 1984; Center for Health Policy Research, *Socioeconomic Characteristics of Medical Practice 1984,* Chicago: American Medical Association, 1984; Daniel Waldo and Helen Lizenby, "Demographic characteristics and health care use and expenditures by the aged in the United States: 1977–1984," *Health Care Financing Review* 6:1–29, 1984; National Center for Health Statistics, *Patients' Reasons for Visiting Physicians: National Ambulatory Medical Care Survey, United States, 1977–78,* DHHS Pub. No. (PHS) 82–1717, 1981; National Center for Health Statistics, *Surgical and Nonsurgical Procedures in Short-Stay Hospitals: United States, 1979,* DHHS Pub. No. (PHS) 83–1731, 1983; National Center for Health Statistics, *The National Nursing Home Survey: 1977 Summary for the United States,* DHHS Pub. No. (PHS) 79–1794, 1979; Eli Ginzberg, "Allied health resources," in David Mechanic (ed.) *Handbook of Health, Health Care, and the Health Profes-*

sions, New York: Free Press, 1983, pp. 479–494; Eugene Levine and Evelyn Moses, "Registered nurses today: a statistical profile," in Linda Aiken (ed.) *Nursing in the 1980's,* Philadelphia: Lippincott, 1982, pp. 475–494; National Center for Health Statistics, Annual Summary of Births, Deaths, Marriages and Divorces: United States, 1983, *Monthly Vital Statistics Report* 32, No. 13, Sept. 21, 1984; American Hospital Association, *Hospital Statistics,* Chicago, 1983; American Hospital Association, *Hospital Statistics,* Chicago, 1984; U.S. General Accounting Office, *Constraining National Health Care Expenditures: Achieving Quality Care at an Affordable Cost,* Sept. 30, 1985.

PART I

Issues in Health Policy

1

Medical Care
and Social Policy

MEDICINE TODAY is dramatically different than just 20 years ago and in a state of innovation and ferment. Advances in medical science and biotechnology have fundamentally altered the processes of medical care, the intensity of hospital work, the mix of health care professionals, and the degree of public and corporate involvement in everyday medical activities. The facts of medical care cost escalation are well known and their detailed recitation unnecessary. Between 1955 and 1983, health care expenditures increased their share of the gross national product from 4.4 to 10.8 per cent, and many expect that even with heroic efforts to hold costs in check, health care may ultimately reach 15 per cent of GNP.

The future of health care in the United States will undoubtedly build on existing forms of organization, traditional professional groupings, and dominant types of facilities, but they are also undergoing significant change. Only by having a strong sense of purpose and direction can we shape significantly emerging patterns in more constructive directions. Many biomedical developments are truly impressive, but the distortions in the total pattern of health care services, and the limited accomplishments for some very large investments, are striking. There is no assurance that careful priorities will prevail over technological imperatives or economic and political pressures, but it is apparent that if we lack a clear conception of our goals, there is not much chance of competing successfully with powerful, persistent, and motivated interest groups. Health care is big business, and those who wish to shape it as a start need a clear vision, well-thought-out strategies, and a great deal of persistence.

In examining the role of health care in a larger context we immediately come upon two inescapable conclusions. First, health is shaped fundamentally by culture, society, and environment and it is mostly at the margins that medical care services have their primary impact. Most of the great advances in health status have come about through basic improvements in economic status, education, nutrition, life-styles, and the environment. Medical care is an important influence, but only one of many. Second, physical and psychological illness, however influenced by inheritance and biology, arise in no small way from conditions in the family, at work, and in the community more generally. Patients' experiences of illness reflect ways of adapting to intolerable stresses that tax their capabilities and spirit as well as their inborn vulnerabilities and noxious agents. The biology and psychology of health are inextricably interconnected.[1]

Medical care, of course, is more narrow than health enhancement, but its goals must be broad. Health care professionals have responsibility to support and sustain those suffering pain, distress, and incapacity and to restore patients to their maximal potential of functioning. Too much of medical care is directed to diagnosis and management of specific diseases and too little to considering how to restore functioning or to assist patients most appropriately within the context of their illnesses and disabilities if cure is elusive. While remarkable progress has been made in the past by pursuing limited concepts of cause and a narrow view of the physician's responsibilities, the changing age profile of the population and prevalent patterns of illness and disability suggest that the challenge for future health professionals will be as much with maintaining function as with cure.

The Role of Physicians and Other Health Professionals

The domain of medicine continues to expand with the medicalization of social problems, and patients come to physicians with a very broad range of complaints. The variety of illnesses presents the physician with responsibilities that require contrasting approaches that may be difficult to negotiate. On the one hand, the specificity of medical knowledge and the sophistication of available technology allow a detailed investigation of complaints and a probable diagnosis. On the other hand, many distressed patients and those with chronic disabilities may require less emphasis on the biological details of their disease and more on techniques of management that facilitate social functioning.

It is accepted that primary care physicians—general internists, pediatricians, and family practitioners—must have broad orientations and skills and the capacity to manage sociomedical problems as well as to deal with disease in a more narrow sense. What is less clear is how physicians, attuned to specific identification of and treatment of conditions based on increasingly sophisticated and focused biological information, can remain alert to the social and emotional implications of how they seek information, how they communicate about treatment, and how they weigh the values and risks of medical interventions against alternative approaches to patient care. The orientations are somewhat antithetical, and by focusing on technical details on some limited aspect of bodily functioning, the probability increases that a view of the whole person will be lost, particularly when physicians work under time pressures. Since detailed clinical knowledge will increase, preparing future physicians to maintain a necessary conception of the whole will be a formidable challenge for medical education.

One approach, promoted in the 1970s, has been the preparation of well-trained generalists, such as the family practitioner or the general internist, who coordinate the necessary subspecialty care on behalf of the patient and who provide longitudinal care and make necessary referrals. This concept of a broad generalist, orchestrating the efforts of a variety of consulting physicians, has great appeal, but it is unlikely to become dominant. Such dominance would call for a majority of generalists with smaller numbers of more specialized physicians, but most physicians are now specialists or subspecialists who keep busy and maintain their incomes by providing general services in addition to specialty care.[2] With the increased numbers of future physicians, and growing competition for patients, it is unlikely that specialists will easily yield much influence and control to a new breed of generalists. A balance of physician manpower is more possible in organized settings such as health maintenance organizations (HMOs), where there are incentives for efficient use of professional personnel. In fee-for-service contexts, the existing reimbursement approaches reinforce subspecialty orientations and the performance of technical procedures in contrast to more time-consuming interviewing, counseling, or education.

Payment mechanisms also affect the use of other health personnel, such as physician assistants, nurse practitioners, and social workers. While there was emphasis in the 1960s and 1970s on enhancing the possibilities of "physician substitution" be developing new health professionals, the present economic climate limits their possibilities unless reimbursement is modified.

With the expansion of the scope of medical practice, and the medicalization of social problems, physicians face new and more complex expectations, many for which they are poorly prepared. Increasingly, the art of medicine is subjected to scientific exploration, making it necessary to treat areas traditionally within the realm of "common sense" with greater knowledge and awareness. The appraisal and diagnosis of psychological disorders have advanced considerably, and both pharmacological and behavioral approaches have become more specific. Physicians, who exclusively treat the vast majority of patients with psychological disorders, are often poorly informed and seriously deficient in the care they provide. Similarly, awareness of and interest in the broad needs of the elderly are limited, and there is a strong tendency in medicine toward excessive technical care while neglecting profound psychosocial and emotional problems.

New expectations leave many physicians somewhat baffled and insecure. Many resent the new regulations and increasing criticisms from patients and fear an erosion of their favored economic status and clinical autonomy. Others, seeing troubles ahead, work to maintain their incomes while conditions allow. Most are groping with approaches that allow them to be responsive to expectations in a framework consistent with their conceptions of how medicine should be practiced and within the constraints imposed by government, insurance companies, hospitals, and their personal needs.

Medical practice in serious illness is inevitably a team effort, involving a variety of physicians, nurses, technicians, and others. As the complexity of the team increases, the possibilities for confusion, lack of coordination, and conflicting efforts mount. There is no alternative to clearly defined responsibility and accountability, and this requires that physicians work jointly with others and share authority. Physicians tend to be individualistic in their orientations and may be inattentive or ineffective as team leaders. Many failures in medical care result from poor coordination and failures in communication among team members. It is simply not sufficient for the physician to be conscientious in the care of the individual patient; if authority is assumed, the physician is responsible as well for the effectiveness of the patient's total care.

Federal Programs in Health

The decade of the 1960s brought massive government involvement in medical care financing and regulation, and one that dramatically altered organizational relationships in health care. The introduction of Medicare and Medicaid in 1966, and its impact on professionals, medical care institutions, and medical care costs, fundamentally changed the relationship between public authorities and private providers. While physicians and institutions benefited immeasurably from the increased financing made available by these programs, they also became quasi-public providers, ceding some of their operating flexibility to external authority.

Massive federal programs contributed to inflation, the overuse of sophisticated but not always necessary technology, and a strong profit orientation in the response of the private sector; however, they also touched the lives of many people in need by providing sophisticated medical care not previously available. Medicare and Medicaid significantly improved access to medical care for elderly persons and for the medically indigent. The traditionally observed relationship between low socioeconomic status and little use of physician services was reversed, and rates of admission to hospitals among the old and disadvantaged increased substantially. In short, these programs brought a better fit between medical need and the accessibility and use of medical resources.

Dramatic improvements in health status coincided with the implementation of Medicare, Medicaid, and other major national programs to eliminate hunger and improve nutrition, protect the health of mothers and children, and to insure accessibility to medical care for disadvantaged groups, through neighborhood health centers and other means. Many factors were involved, but clearly these programs had an important role in improving health. In the mid-1950s, length of life in the United States stabilized and in the following decade changed little. Beginning in the mid-1960s, age-specific death rates began to decline, substantially increasing life expectancy, with significant gains particularly for the elderly population. In 1983, life expectancy at birth almost reached 75 years—79 years for white women.[3] Even more impressive is that these advances do not appear to be associated with significant increases in disability.[4] Old people at all ages appear to be healthier than ever before, often advancing well into old age before experiencing significant debility. Infant mortality also declined from 20.9 in 1968–1970 to 10.9 in 1983. Large improvements are evident among both whites and nonwhites, but the gap between the races has continued. Black infant mortality remains almost double that of whites, and blacks continue to lag well behind the white population in longevity.

In 1983, government at all levels contributed almost 42 per cent of total health expenditures, $148.8 billion, of which $57.4 billion was for Medicare and $34 billion for Medicaid. The Medicare Hospital Trust Fund, consisting of payroll tax revenues, is expected to be depleted by the late 1990s, and Medicaid's burden on state budgets has already resulted in significant reductions in eligibility and benefits. Concern for the poor is now overshadowed by the large aggregate costs of these programs, by the growing federal deficit, and by the need to restrain medical care costs more generally. In this context of conflicting needs and pressures, cost containment has become the biggest game in town.

The Changing Medical Care Arena

In broad terms, two major ideological approaches have dominated discussions of health affairs in the United States. The first, a planning or regulatory perspective, is based on the assumption that health resources can be allocated best through needs assessment and shaping access and entitlement in relation to expert judgment. A competing view is that patients, and organizations that are large purchasers of care, allowed to exercise their own judgment in a competitive marketplace will introduce a more efficient and effective pattern of care than one determined and regulated by government authorities.[5] Neither ideology accurately depicts the complexity and diversity of the health field nor the socioeconomic, political, and behavioral barriers to any monolithic solution, whether based on competition or planning.

The adequate provision of care depends on appropriate personnel and facilities, financing, suitable organizational forms for delivering services, and means of maintaining and assuring quality of care. Each of these areas has been an important focus of public concern and social policy. In the manpower area, for example, federal policy has been a major factor. By the late 1950s, it had become evident that newly trained physicians were not replacing retiring general practitioners either in relation to types of functions performed or in the geographic location of their practices. There was growing concern about the unavailability of physicians, particularly generalists. The problem, as conceptualized in the decade of the 1960s, was one of a doctor shortage, and the prevalent belief was that with adequate numbers, market forces would produce better specialty balance and geographic dispersion.

The approach of government was to encourage the development of new medical schools and to provide financial incentives in the form of capitation payments to existing schools to increase enrollment. Initially, there was great reluctance to interfere with medical education beyond providing financial incentives for growth; however, over time, capitation was targeted more specifically to achieve social objectives such as closing the gap between primary care and specialty practice. Government policy, even when more focused, avoided direct intervention into educational affairs and, thus, had to approach policy goals on the assumption that geographic dispersion and specialty balance would result from an increase in medical manpower.[6] While the focus of manpower policy was physicians, efforts were made on many fronts to increase primary care personnel with government subsidization of the training of nurses, nurse practitioners, physician assistants, mental health professionals, and many others.

Government was remarkably successful in its basic goal to increase health care manpower. The output of American medical schools was doubled, and supporting health personnel were educated in large numbers. In retrospect, our successes have introduced new and substantial problems. While there is some evidence that, with the growth of manpower, market forces work toward some redistribution,[7] in actuality it occurs only very slowly. As economic conditions have altered, the large impending physician excess projected in the next decade[8] seems to some more ominous than the problems growth was intended to solve. We have learned some hard lessons: that with growing numbers of doctors, fees are not necessarily reduced; that each physician generates costs far greater than the expense of his or her own remuneration; and that professionals have considerable discretion in determining medical necessity in uncertain circumstances and, thus, have at least partial control over demand for their services. All of these factors helped insulate physicians against economic forces, with fee-for-service third-party insurance constituting the key protection by diluting the impact of cost felt by the public.

The growth of investment in health care has spawned major industries with billions of dollars of profit at stake. Most remarkable, perhaps, is the rapid growth of multihospital corporations, proprietary nursing homes, freestanding hemodialysis units, surgi-centers, diagnostic laboratories, and for-profit home care and emergency services among others. Arnold Relman, editor of the *New England Journal of Medicine*, in bringing the growth of this commercialized activity to the attention of the medical community, dubbed it "the new medical-industrial complex," in contrast to the more traditional industries manufacturing pharmaceutical and medical equipment supplies.[9] He defines this new complex as "a large and growing network of private corporations engaged in the business of supplying health-care services to patients for a profit—services heretofore provided by nonprofit institutions or individual practitioners" (p. 963). He estimated that in 1979 such profit-oriented activities yielded a gross of $35 to $40 billion. Other strong interests include the nonprofit hospital industry, medical and other professional groups, the medical schools and teaching hospitals, profit and nonprofit intermediaries who administer vast government and other expenditures, and a variety of disease lobbies. It should be plain that health policy is more politicized than ever before, and that future problems must be resolved in an extraordinarily complex arena.

The number of hospitals has remained stable in recent years, but the complexity of their technologies and personnel needs has altered fundamentally. The focus of growing regulatory activity in hospitals is cost containment, and the concern is to minimize unnecessary utilization, reduce bed capacity, and control the expansion of sophisticated and expensive technologies. While there has been uneven success, hospitals have become more cost conscious in response to the risk of having reimbursement disallowed. In recent years, there has been an influx of hospital administrators better versed in financing and managerial functions but not always sensitive to the consequences of administrative decisions for patient care.

The entry of large-scale proprietary health care interests on the one hand and tougher cost-containment efforts by government and other third parties on the other has thrown the hospital sector into disarray. For-profit chains seek public legitimacy and physician acceptance and often make gestures at community involvement and technological superiority, such as Humana's large and highly visible decision to transplant 100 artificial hearts. The voluntary sector, facing a more competitive environment, is increasingly hedging its bets by spinning off profit-oriented subsidiaries. As both types of hospitals jockey for position in future health care markets, they may become increasingly difficult to differentiate. The public hospital, in contrast, finds itself with larger numbers of sick poor and difficult multiproblem patients, covered by Medicaid or without insurance, that other sectors seek to avoid, and an erosion of public commitment to insuring that they have the capacity to maintain decent levels of care.[10]

The psychology of illness, and the importance that consumers give to their own medical care, also contribute to the difficulty of policy formulation. Reasonable consumers can see the logic of more efficient distribution and organization of services, more parsimonious use of laboratories and technologies, and allocating resources in some relation to expected benefits, but when sick they want the best that medical science makes possible, and these wants are reinforced under a third-party payment system. While most people agree, in principle, that excess hospital beds should be eliminated or converted to other uses, in practice they want the principle to apply only to other people's hospitals. There is agreement that frivolous utilization and expenditures should be discouraged, but few patients ever think their own problems frivolous or unworthy of the best care available.

Responses to Cost Pressures

There have been a great variety of responses to rising costs reflecting
the impact on employers, institutions, and federal and state budgets.
Although there has been a great deal of rhetoric about competition
in health, and some modest progress in encouraging alternative health
systems and more sophisticated purchasing of health insurance
among large buyers, most of the activity thus far is better described
as costshifting and regulation.

In the public sector, eligibility has been much more strictly limited in the Medicaid program, and co-insurance, deductibles, and
premiums have been increased among Medicare recipients. Further
limitations continue under consideration.[11] The federal government
has also frozen physician payment for specified periods under Medicare, more strictly limited hospital reimbursement, and recently introduced reimbursement by diagnosis-related groups (DRGs), which
pays hospitals a flat amount based on the patients' diagnostic classification as compared to paying the hospital its actual charges.
Peer review organizations have been mandated to more strictly review hospital utilization and surgical admissions. The federal government also has made program changes to facilitate the enrollment of
Medicare recipients in health maintenance organizations.

States have adopted a variety of cost-control efforts. Some
states—for example, California, Wisconsin, and Arizona—have
contracted with preferred provider organizations that serve recipients receiving state aid at prenegotiated prices. In New York, Massachusetts, and other states, tough rate regulation and controls on
new capital investment have required the hospital sector to change
its traditional modes of operation and management. New Jersey
maintains a DRG system, somewhat different than the Medicare system, that applies to all payers and not solely to the Medicare program. It is still too early to clearly assess how effectively these
alternative approaches control aggregate costs.

In the private sector, major employers, who have faced escalating
medical fringe benefit costs for some years, have reacted to mounting costs by self-insuring their employees, by establishing their own
health care plans, by providing economic inducements to employees
to use less medical care, and by imposing greater cost-sharing requirements on employee health insurance coverage. One study found

that major employers requiring hospital deductibles increased from 30 to 63 per cent between 1982 and 1984.[12]

Technological Imperatives and the Effects of Distorted Incentives

The challenges of the 1980s and beyond are made difficult not only by economic constraints but also by changing definitions of the content of medical care consistent with technological advances. Medical care quickly incorporates the latest advances in biomedical technology, sometimes increasing new possibilities for maintaining life and preserving function, but often adding new increments of cost without clear benefits. The expansion of neonatal intensive care reflects the impressive capacity of acute care medicine in implementing life-saving technologies. We now invest relatively large resources to save babies of increasingly lower birth weights. The Office of Technology Assessment estimated that $1.5 billion was spent on neonatal intensive care in 1978. Average cost per case was approximately $8,000. These costs have continued to increase, particularly as the technology is applied to smaller and smaller infants whose survival is highly uncertain. A small number of these babies whose defects render them ventilator dependent may spend years in the hospital following birth at costs approaching a million dollars. Average duration of intensive care for such babies has been estimated to be from 200 to 500 days.[13]

High technology comes into play again at the end of life, where heroic technologies are often applied to delay death for a short time. In 1980, the 11 per cent of persons overt 65 accounted for 31 per cent of health expenditures.[14] While this in itself is not surprising since the elderly have more illness and need more care than younger groups, much of these expenditures occur in the last year of life, and of these costs, almost half occur in the two months prior to death. It is obviously difficult to anticipate who will live and who will die, but there is substantial agreement that heroic technology at the end of life does not use available resources to maximize the social welfare of the elderly. The resolution of these difficult issues remain unclear. It is apparent, however, that demographic changes will put increased pressure on the Medicaid program as well as Medicare in future years, or on whatever alternative long-term care programs we develop.

The increasing use of halfway technologies for middle-aged populations also raises immense issues. Coronary bypass surgery has become increasingly routine; 170,000 operations were performed in 1982 at a cost of $2.5 billion. This operation, in contrast to more conservative medical treatment, preserves life only in disease of the left main coronary artery or when there is extensive atheroslerosis in three sites in the coronary arteries. In other instances it reduces pain and can be justified as well on that basis. But frequently it is undertaken despite its lack of superiority to medical treatment. Many of these operations may ultimately be replaced by angioplasty, a more simple surgical procedure in which a balloon catheter is used to unblock arteries. If this procedure proves to be effective, it will probably reduce the growing prevalence of bypass surgery, but it is subject to similar potential abuse. Similarly, coronary intensive care at a very high cost has become routine for treatment of heart attacks although the evidence fails to support its value relative to more conventional care.[15] We are now beginning a new era in heart transplantation with the success of the immunosuppressive drug Cyclosporine, the accelerated efforts in transplantation of mechanical hearts, and partial heart replacements as well. Liver transplantation is now viable and is covered by many health insurance programs. It is inevitable that these technologies will be perfected increasingly, and will confront us with difficult social choices.

A dramatic but instructive example of the imperatives of technology is the End-Stage Renal Disease Program. In he mid-1960s, approximately 1,000 patients were on dialysis, but it was estimated that as many as 6,000 patients died because of the lack of available resources.[9] In 1972, a vigorous lobby on behalf of kidney disease victims was successful in obtaining categorical legislation covering patients with chronic renal disease under Medicare. Dialysis facilities proliferated following the legislation, and now proprietary units provide approximately 40 per cent of all hemodialysis treatment. In 1983, 63,000 patients were estimated to be on dialysis, covered by Medicare, at a cost of approximately $2 billion. While in many instances hemodialysis is a lifesaving procedure that allows the patient to continue at a reasonable level of functioning, existing incentives encourage treatment even when little life of quality may remain.

The number of such new technologies will proliferate in the future, and as it becomes less possible to provide all the alternatives that medical science offers, we will be faced with tough choices. It will become more difficult to use expensive technologies simply because they offer some small possibility of advantage; their use will have to be weighed against alternative uses of finite resources.

The Dilemmas of Regulation

Medicine in the United States is highly regulated and is increasingly bureaucratized. This trend affects not only all institutional providers but also smaller medical care practices, even the individual office-based physician. American doctors are more highly monitored and regulated than doctors in many other countries, despite the strong ideology concerning the autonomy and freedom of the physician. Such regulation comes from all units of government, reimbursement programs, and private professional groups. American doctors are significantly more burdened with detailed rules and guidelines relating to their modes of practice and clinical work than their English counterparts, although the latter are generally believed to be under more stringent control. While the English administratively establish general constraints on the economics of care, they intervene less at the level of patient care than we do. Physician regulation in the United States is very extensive and applied in a way that is costly and burdensome. The need to maintain the mirage of a private sector of medical care in the United States, I believe, results in consequences opposite to those desired—a rather heavy hand of government on the process of medical care. Despite its rhetoric, the Reagan program has instituted tougher medical care regulations than most previous administrations.

Medical bureaucracy in the United States arises from sources other than the technical complexity of sophisticated medical care. First is the need to reimburse, on an individual fee-for-service or a cost-reimbursement basis, large numbers of professionals and organizational providers, and to audit bills consistent with regulations. The billing process itself, and the paperwork necessary to monitor numerous and complex third-party insurance contracts—with varying eligibility criteria, co-insurance, deductibles, and maximum benefit schedules and with widely varying coverage and criteria for major medical payments—boggles the mind and would have been impossible without the development of sophisticated computer systems. Although this complexity may serve insurance companies in preventing consumer comparisons, it assuredly confuses both patients and their doctors. In the case of professionals and institutions, the complexity of billing procedures and the cash flow of third-party reimbursement are often significant problems.

Government involvement in medical care also comes not through a few broad strokes but rather through hundreds of programs and thousands of guidelines and special criteria. Each program developed to attack some special categorical or administrative concern has its own specifications, conditions for eligibility, and administrative guidelines. In each instance the specific criteria and guidelines promulgated can be justified, but in the aggregate they often work at cross-purposes, and the cost involved in monitoring and compliance can be staggering. The prevalent perspective is that rules are salutory, and little consideration is given to matching up the benefits with the costs of new regulatory activity. Rules proliferate at a rapid rate, are frequently unenforceable, and government often lacks the capacity to monitor seriously. The result is that organizations become adept at manipulating definitions, budgets, and procedures, and even the most important requirements are commonly subverted. The proliferation of trivia often diverts attention from the really important issues.

Although it might be argued that the United States has followed a middle course between the harsh realities of a private medical marketplace, and a highly regulated system, this is more illusion than reality. The middle course is costly and inefficient in its administrative demands while offering less real protection to the public than is generally assumed. As each new problem surfaces, new rules are designed to confront the problem. In any individual case, the rules, although often indirect to deflate strong opposition among those being regulated, have some rationale and justification. The total pattern of regulatory activity, however, is a crazy quilt of rules that often operate at cross-purposes, require considerable resources of time and money, and undermine morale and vitality. Within institutions, it shifts power from those who provide care to financial and administrative personnel whose responsibility it is to insure compliance and who monitor activities consistent with existing legislation and procedures.

It is clear that regulation is an essential aspect of large-scale organization. Rules are attempts to specify how activities are to be carried out and are intended to substitute for protracted and acrimonious interpersonal negotiation. One approach to rule-making is to establish standards as each problem arises, on the assumption that direction is needed. An alternative is to view regulation as an activity carrying both potential benefits and costs. Before new rules are imposed, it becomes necessary to calculate the trade-offs between what one achieves with a rule and the cost of imposing it on the various parties affected.

A related issue is the level at which it is most appropriate for administrative authority to be applied. Certainly, central government has the informational resources to make economic and organizational calculations to define broad principles and necessary constraints. Centralized authority, however, has great difficulty in successfully monitoring, or even understanding, the complexities and contingencies at the level of patient care, and intrusions into these areas often have perverse consequences. Moreover, when the inflexibility and inappropriateness of specific guidelines are experienced by those affected, the result is often not only a subversion of central authority but also, and even more important, a loss of its legitimacy. Effective regulation, thus, is restrained. It sets constraints but delegates specific decisions to those who are responsible for delivering the necessary services and know the immediate facts.

Alternatives to the Regulatory Muddle

There are basically two radical alternatives to the proliferation of government rule-making. The first encourages a private market within specified boundaries but with minimal detailed interference. The second builds on prospective budgeting to health providers who take responsibility for the needs of defined populations. Although the range of services and coverage is mandated, the health care unit itself has great discretion in the establishment of procedures, priorities, and resource allocations. In each case, government sets the framework but remains detached from the day-to-day operations of medical care.

The private marketplace is a radical alternative because such a marketplace does not exist and would be difficult to establish. Although the price and responsiveness of some types of medical programs and services are favorably influenced by more competition—e.g., the structure of medical insurance plans, the cost of drugs and

medical devices, or even the fees for particular surgical procedures—
the core aspect of medical care, involving the physician's assessment
of patients' complaints and the sequence of decision-making and
treatment, is not likely to be much affected by the presence of a more
competitive marketplace. Yet this is the essence of the medical care
process and the aspect of care of greatest concern to both patients
and physicians.

Proponents see the marketplace approach as the best means of
maximizing allocative efficiency and believe that any major problems of equity can be approached through selective subsidy or income redistribution. Stimulating the marketplace, they believe,
requires considerable deregulation of professional controls, encouragement of advertising, and stimulation of consumer power in deciding the allocations of their medical dollars. Government subsidy
would come in the form of economic entitlements that the consumer
could exchange for varying types of insurance plans. Thus incentives
would exist to encourage more economical choices; patients would
share in the costs or benefits when they selected more or less expensive medical alternatives. While government might set boundaries and
constraints on what trade-offs take place in the system to avoid catastrophic situations that consumers fail to anticipate, consumers
would have considerable discretion as to the type and amount of
services they purchase beyond a standard minimum, and thus what
the cost would be to them. Under Enthoven's well-known pro-
posal,[16] for example, consumers would have a subsidy to purchase
varying insurance policies meeting established minimum standards,
but then could add amenities or not, depending on their personal
inclinations and circumstances.

The marketplace models assume responsiveness of the institutional sector (including health insurance plans, hospitals, and professionals) to the new economic climate, but there is at best only modest
evidence that the types of responsiveness envisioned would actually
occur. One must assume that the consumers would make informed
economic choices on the basis of economic interests rather than habit,
inertia, or psychological considerations, and that large providers
would feel pressured to compete in offering more economical and
efficient plans. One must also assume that such providers have and
could use their institutional powers to effectively constrain physician
decision-making. Although the theory has a certain plausibility, it
depends on many uncertain assumptions and a radical restructuring

of existing institutional arrangements and practice patterns. It would certainly require a great deal of momentum to get there from where we are at present.

The alternative approach, more consistent with existing organization if not with prevalent social ideologies, is to put increasing economic constraints on the medical sector, creating pressures for professionals and organizational providers to establish new priorities and operating procedures. Payments could come in the form of capitation or negotiated budgets. In contrast to explicit mandates on how funds could be expended and for what purposes, each service program would be encouraged to assess its responsibilities and priorities for meeting them. In short, autonomy would be protected but in a constraining environment in which efficiencies would be required.

How is the public to be assured that their needs will be met, however? How can access to entitlements, sensitive and responsive care, and a willingness to treat patients equitably be enforced? Only the naive would assume that medical institutions and professionals under pressure would necessarily come to decisions in the public's interest, particularly when the public interest may be in opposition to their own. Yet we know from present experience how difficult it is to regulate relationships between medical institutions, professionals, and patients, and what a costly burden these regulatory activities can be for all concerned.

There is no optimal solution to such issues, only varying imperfect options that will be discussed throughout this book. Any system in which patients are linked with particular providers on a capitation or budgetary basis should provide as much patient choice as possible, and make it simple for patients to shift providers easily and with relatively short notice. While this may create some administrative burdens and instability of financing, the organizations and providers most affected would be those with the most dissatisfied patients. Formal structural support for consumer choice increases the possibilities for countervailing influence relative to the immense power of professionals and organizations. Such influence is maximized when information about providers is readily available and can be disseminated easily. Individual consumers typically do not have the resources to obtain adequate information, but representatives of consumers, such as union welfare funds, consumer organizations, or even official groups, state insurance departments for example, might be encouraged to play a larger role in bringing pertinent considerations and performance data to the attention of constituents. The Health Care Financing Administration (HCFA), which administers Medicare, is planning to give consumers access to information on such indicators as mortality rate by hospital for varying surgical procedures, number of patients developing postoperative infections, average length of hospital stay, and cost and volume of various procedures performed at each hospital. As consumer organizations become more expert in monitoring medical services, they might develop considerable bargaining power to affect provider priorities and practices.

It is difficult to be complacent about the possibilities of constructive change in a context so complicated, so fettered with entrenched traditions and interests, and so perverse in existing incentives. Pressures on the federal budget and on costs more generally, however, have produced a need for readjustment and provides an opportunity to reshape in some major ways the conditions affecting practice. There is a consensus on two points: that costs must be brought under better control, and that regulation is a burden. A constructive strategy overall is to plan to reduce regulatory pressures as the health sector demonstrates a willingness to work within a more controllable reimbursement policy and to take responsibility for developing internal processes of accountability consistent with concern for reasonable access, quality, and equity.

References

1. Mechanic D. Medical sociology, 2d ed. New York: Free Press, 1978.
2. Aiken L, et al. The contribution of specialists to the delivery of primary care. N Engl J Med. 1979; 300:1363–1370.
3. National Center for Health Statistics. Monthly vital statistics report 32. Hyattsville, Md.: National Center for Health Statistics, 1984. (DHHS publication no. [PHS] 84–1120.)
4. Fuchs V. "Though much is taken": reflections on aging, health and medical care. Health Soc. 1984; 62:143–166.
5. Enthoven A. The competition strategy: status and prospects. N Engl J Med. 1981; 304:109–112.
6. Lewis CE, Fein R, Mechanic D. A right to health: the problem of access to primary medical care. New York: Wiley-Interscience, 1976.
7. Schwartz W, Newhouse J, Bennett B, et al. The changing geographic

distribution of board-certified physicians. N Engl J Med. 1980; 303:1032–1038.

8. Health Resources Administration. Health resource news 7. Washington, D.C.: Health Resources Administration, 1980.

9. Relman AS. The new medical-industrial complex. N Engl J Med. 1980; 303:963–970.

10. Hadley J, Feder J. Troubled hospitals: poor patients or management? Bus Health. 1984; 1:15–19.

11. Aiken L, Bays K. The Medicare debate—round one. N Engl J Med. 1984; 311:1196–1200.

12. Hewitt and Associates. Company practices in health care management. Lincolnshire, Ill.: Hewitt and Associates, 1984.

13. U.S. Department of Health and Human Services. Report of the surgeon general's workshop on children with handicaps and their families. Hyattsville, Md.: National Center for Health Statistics, 1982. (DHHS publication no. 83-50194:12.)

14. U.S. Department of Health and Human Services. Health—United States, 1983. Washngton, D.C.: National Center for Health Statistics, 1984. (DHHS publication no. [PHS] 84-1232:146-147.)

15. Waitzkin H. A marxian interpretation of the growth and development of coronary care technology. Amer J Pub Health. 1979; 69:1260–1268.

16. Enthoven A. Health plan: the only practical solution to the soaring cost of medical care. Reading, Mass.: Addison-Wesley, 1980.

2

Approaches to Controlling Medical Care Costs

THE CONCEPT OF RATIONING MEDICAL CARE has an odious ring to many ears, but rationing of care has always been the norm in the United States and elsewhere.[1] No community has ever provided all the care that its population might be willing to use, and the magnitude of consumption has reflected the manpower and facilites available, the price of services and the noneconomic barriers to care such as queues, waiting time, and distance to sites of care. An important change, however, is the extent to which services are free of cost or limited to the recipient at the point of consumption. As government and third parties have come to cover an increasing proportion of medical care costs, there have been fewer financial inhibitions on the use of services. Thus, the marketplace as a rationing process increasingly has been replaced by consciously planned means of rationing either by government edict or through incentives or controls intended to change the behavior of health professionals.

Rationing is simply a means to apportion or distribute some good through a method of allowance. As the marketplace becomes a less important method of allowance, the mix of cost-containment techniques changes. The agenda is to understand better what a good mix is, not only from the perspective of achieving economies, but also to improve quality, enhance interactions between health professionals and patients, and to provide opportunities for trust and mutual respect. More stringent rationing must also be weighed against alternative strategies that either change the dependence of the population on the physician and its demands for more medical care, that improve the production of medical services, or that develop alternative community structures to deal with many types of problems typically treated by physicians.

Factors Affecting the Consumption of Services

A major way to reduce expenditures for medical care and the requirement for developing more facilities and personnel is to limit the needs and desires among patients for medical care. Reducing needs involves the prevention of illness or diminishing patients' psychological dependence on the medical encounter for social support or other secondary advantages. Reducing desire for services requires changing people's views of the value of different types of medical care, making them more aware of the real costs of service in relation to the benefits received, and legitimizing alternatives for dealing with many problems that physicians increasingly deal with as the boundaries of medical care expand.

Prevention can be conceived of broadly as having three aspects. At the most global level are efforts in sectors other than health affecting the quality of the environment: standards of living, education, and nutrition; employment; and other social conditions relevant to health status.[2] The benefits of pollution control, for example, in relation to cost are high, and such efforts add to health status, by reducing prevalence of disease, as well as to the quality of living.[3] Possibilities for preventive efforts outside the medical sector are considerable, but the required policies frequently compete with economic and other social priorities and may be difficult to implement.

A second approach to prevention involves clearly identifying risk factors and structuring the environment or motivating people to minimize them. Although the examples of cigarette smoking, alcohol and drug dependence, and inactivity and obesity are most frequently cited, these are complex behavioral problems that do not yield simply to exhortation or educational approaches. Often, these behaviors are deeply rooted in personality and are related to other serious problems that are intractable to change. Although there is sufficient evidence of progress in changing the population's habits to avoid excessive pessimism[4] it is prudent to recognize the difficulty of the task, the forces working against successful change, and the depths of ignorance concerning the origins of these behaviors and the ways in which they can best be modified. It may be that the greatest potential in changing health behavior is by focusing on the young before these behavioral patterns become well entrenched, but overcoming the influence of peer groups and other incentives to dangerous habits remains a formidable task.

A complementary approach is to make efforts to design living environments that reduce risk regardless of individual behavior.[5] The inflatable airbag in automobiles, fortified food, and the safe cigarette are examples. Moreover, daily routine patterns of healthful behavior such as exercise[6] can be introduced into social environments in which persons spend much of their time, such as the workplace. Although technologic alternatives to changing individual behavior have been vigorously advocated, a prudent social policy would direct efforts to both behavior change and technologic alternatives. Too great an emphasis on technology alone might create disincentives for young people to develop responsible behavior relevant to their health.

Closest to the delivery of medical services are primary prevention programs such as immunization and early screening and treatment of disease and disabilities. In such areas as control of hypertension, effective diagnosis and treatment are available, but overcoming the behaviorial problem of achieving continuing cooperation still constitutes a major barrier. Early detection of vision and hearing difficulties also limits later problems and costs and does not involve major behavioral barriers. Appropriate treatment of common childhood ailments such as streptococcal infections and otitis media avoid damaging secondary problems that may result in the consumption of considerable services in adult life.[7] The difficulty is that beyond a limited number of instances, preventive or early care remains an untested concept, and the costs of identifying a small number of cases of asymptomatic illness early may be prohibitive.[8] To the extent that nontreatable asymptomatic disease is detected and made known to the patient, the consequences may be counterproductive because of the anxiety and worry aroused, socially induced disability, or stigmatization.

Another way of reducing demand for care to to modify patients' perceptions of its value or appropriateness. There seems to be a consensus that patients have exceptionally high and unrealistic expectations of physicians and that they become too dependent on medical care. A number of studies have found that unrealistic expectations result in disappointment and less successful outcomes.[9] Although the medical profession may have contributed to such excessive expectations by exaggerating the effects of medical advances, it is in the interests of both patients and physicians to have the public better informed about the limitations of medical care as well as its benefits. The challenge is to educate the patient without encouraging further distrust of physicians and their work.

Changing expectations is an exercise in modifying the culture of medical care. This process requires changing perceptions of how particular health and illness incidents are to be handled, and such modified conceptions may involve as much adjustment for the physician as for the patient. Extreme examples are the redefinition of the appropriate way to die and the development of hospices, with many preferring a less frantic end in the company of their loved ones and sympathetic health personnel to the stupor and high technology associated with the intensive-care unit. The growth of technology has shaped services to a larger degree than patients' needs or desires or prudent expenditure patterns would justify. Third-party payment has made it possible to finance new technology without tough consideration of whether its benefits outweigh its costs. Cultural redefinitions would encourage patients to demand different ways of dealing with many problems.

As patients become better educated about the value, but also about the risks and limitations, of many medical procedures, they may be less likely to demand dangerous interventions that are unnecessary. Mothers may become less enthusiastic about tonsilectomies and routine x-ray studies, and patients with ordinary colds, weight problems, and insominia less demanding of drugs. Moreover, as patients become better informed less responsible physicians will have greater difficulties in carrying out inappropriate procedures and treatments. The task is fairly subtle, and the challenge is to teach patients to question constructively and physicians to respond to such questioning appropriately and in a manner that builds on the patient's trust in the physician's competence and good intentions.

Factors Affecting the Production of Services

In recent years, there has been much attention on the training of physician assistants and nurse practitioners, to the development of health maintenance organizations, and to improved information systems and managerial practices. These may all be ways to increase efficiency in the production of services. Medical care in Western countries is dependent on advanced technologies and expensive personnel. The ordinary medical encounter depends less on communication and clinical judgment and increasingly more on a battery of expensive diagnostic procedures and laboratory tests. The bias in medical care is toward what Fuchs has called the technologic imperative[10]—a tendency to take action, whatever the cost, if it offers even a slight possibility of utility. This situation increases the costs of medical care without evidence that the benefits exceed those of adopting a modest approach.

Methods of production refer to the way in which problems are handled, the time devoted to each case, the routine procedures performed, and the apportionment of tasks among personnel. For example, one Kaiser plan provides a multiphasic health examination performed largely by technicians as a substitute for the more traditional annual examination performed almost exclusively by physicians. Also, clinicians and clinics may vary in the amount of time that they schedule for new and routine visits, the procedures conventionally performed with new patients and modes of dealing with routine problems. Production of services may be affected in four ways: by changing the mix of personnel involved; by changing the technologic inputs; by changing the content of the encounter; or by changing the auspices of care. For example, nurse practitioners can substitute for physicians quite successfully for certain types of care, as a variety of studies have demonstrated,[11] and many aspects of care can be transferred to nurses, physician assistants, and others in a way that improves the productivity of the physician.[12] Similarly, specialists and subspecialists in primary care settings order more procedures than family physicians and general practitioners and have longer encounters.[13] Although such production methods may involve higher quality, the benefits derived from a more intensive technical approach in ambulatory settings remain conjectural.[14] The use of laboratory and many other diagnostic and technical aids can be contained not only to reduce cost and limit iatrogenic diseases but also to improve the quality of care.[15] Shifting the auspices of care may involve considerable economics as well. Hospital-based care for a particular problem is almost always more expensive, and ambulatory hospital-based practices may use more procedures than freestanding practices and thus increase the costs of care. For hospital care, studies in relation to a wide variety of conditions suggest that length of stay can be reduced without any demonstrable medical consequences.

There is a compelling need for investigation of the relation between production methods and patient outcome. Although there is an implicit bias in medical practice that more is better, alternative production methods that devote time to knowing the patient and communicating effectively may yield more valuable results than increasing the intensity of technology. When the "art of medicine" and social care are considered, the role of functional alternatives becomes more obvious.

Functional Alternatives to Existing Medical Care Patterns

Developments in medical technology, unless of a preventive type such as immunization, tend to increase the costs of a typical medical encounter. As more is known and as more can be done, patients' expectations increase, and they demand increased coverage for medical care. To facilitate the effective use of physician resources, it is desirable to shift to other sectors to the extent possible the services that nonprofessionals and other types of professionals can provide as well and at less cost.

Although estimates vary depending on the criteria used, there is agreement from both clinical judgments and the epidemiologic evidence that much of the demand for medical care arises from conditions that physicians are powerless to change or that are simple in terms of the kinds of care required.[16] The utilization of medical care is influenced by illness behavior[17]—the varied ways in which persons identify, define, and evaluate symptoms and what to do about them. Three modes of illness behavior are most relevant here. The first consists of many patients with common self-limited problems that may cause discomfort for a short time but little harm and in any case are not amenable to effective medical intervention. The second are a large variety of minor complaints that can be treated successfully but in which self-care can serve as a suitable substitute with modest self-care aids. The third, and most problematic, are the relatively large numbers of patients with mild and moderate depressions, anxiety, psychosomatic discomforts, and insomnia who frequently come to physicians seeking relief of distress, support, and reassurance. Epidemiologic surveys suggest that at any given time approximately one-fifth of the population may be characterized in this way. Those that come to physicians may be truly suffering, but the hurried and technical stance of the physician in busy ambulatory settings may contribute little to providing the support and comfort that these patients require. The problem of care is made even more difficult because these patients do not explicitly acknowledge the nature of their discomforts, mask these problems with presentations of vague physical symptoms, and often resist psychologic redefinitions of their distress.[18]

Athough physicians must continue to deal with many of these problems and must do so more capably, alternatives exist through development of self-help groups, improved community networks of social support, and a variety of voluntary and professional counseling and information services. To the extent that such services are developed, are defined as legitimate, and avoid excessive professionalization of personnel, they are likely to reach more people at lower cost than the current medical care structure. However, because many such problems will continue to be first recognized through the medical care system, physicians must learn to work cooperatively with other helping services and make referrals to them. Opportunities for linking self-help and other community helping services to the mainstream of medical care will vary with the reimbursement system.

A model that is instructive is Planned Parenthood. Although the provision of contraceptive services has been seen as a medical function, and physicians continue to do a great deal in this area, many persons are not effectively reached through the medical sector. Planned Parenthood clinics, staffed largely by nonphysicians, reach many needy people, providing them with levels of assistance and instruction often unavailable from busy physicians. More time may be given to each client for careful instruction, questioning, and feedback.

Care for the elderly is an area with large potential for alternative types of service. Old people inevitably have chronic illness, and the financing structure encourages a reliance on medical and particularly hospital care. Medicare has brought many benefits to old people who have serious medical problems that require and can benefit from appropriate interventions. But simple social measures that contribute to the continued participation of the elderly and to a sense of meaningful activity can often do more to promote their well-being than narrow technical interventions. Perceived health among the elderly is less positive among persons with a history of depression, who feel neglected and whose morale is low,[19] and self-ratings of health are the strongest correlate of life satisfaction among old people.[20] Medical practice has also become entirely too dependent on total institutional care for old people. Although this development is a product of other trends in the society, existing social policies do little to facilitate the encouragement of independence and continued community functioning among the old. The type of "institutionalism" characteristic of many nursing homes is destructive of human morale,[21] and such facilities should surely be the last resource.

Although this discussion is focused on theoretical options, it is prudent to remain aware that medical care is one of the largest industries, and large sectors of the population depend on it for their employment.[22] Any change in the direction of medical care must be accomplished by retraining of health workers for a variety of new functions such as helping persons to remain in community housing and to function at their highest possible level, providing homemaker services and supervising activity, exercise, and recreation. Employees, through their unions, have increasingly used their political leverage to oppose the closing of institutions or the merger of services. Efforts to revise priorities will require widespread cooperation, community commitment, and wise planning.

The Role of the Health Sciences

Most of the alternatives for cost containment in the long run depend on the acquisition of basic and applied knowledge that identifies causes and effective interventions in disease, that facilitates community prevention and behavior modification, and that provides information on how the medical care system is working and how its quality and efficiency can be improved. The causes of most major diseases remain unknown, and efforts are mostly ameliorative. Halfway technologies, as Lewis Thomas[23] has noted, are enormously expensive in relation to the uncertain results achieved. The future depends on improved basic knowledge that promotes primary prevention and more targeted treatments.

In the behavioral field, much rhetoric is devoted to the ideas of responsibility for health and self-care. The patterns of behavior, however, that require modification are complex responses that have their roots in social and economic patterns, in values and aspirations, modes of socializing the young, peer influence and the mass media, and in many other factors that are only poorly understood. Although society seems prepared to rush ahead with large-scale programs, it seems less willing to invest in the rigorous research necessary that will give a better understanding of the behaviors that should be changed and the ways in which they might successfully be modified. The questions are numerous. To cite some examples: Is clinical depression related to patterns of learned helplessness, and can such patterns be unlearned? Can biofeedback be used to facilitate self-regulation of noxious physiologic states, and what long-term effect can it have on the occurrence of illness and disability? Does the modification of Type-A behavior traits associated with coronary heart disease affect the occurrence of disease or its course? What types of psychologic and social management best contain disability associated with chronic disease, and how can social supports prevent secondary disability often associated with illness?

Health-services research, in contrast, focuses on the organization, financing, and quality of care.[24] It deals with questions of distribution of care, access to care, and outcomes. It evaluates the consequences resulting from innovations in health personnel, new technologies, and modified ways of delivering care. It examines the costs and benefits of various alternatives and the manner in which new practices are adopted and implemented. It studies the effects of different patterns of remuneration on physicians and varying incentives and cost-sharing obligations on patients. In short, health-services research deals with many of the issues reviewed that remain problematic and require further conceptualization and inquiry.

References

1. Mechanic D. The growth of medical technology and bureaucracy: implications for medical care. Health Soc: Milbank Mem Fund Quar. 1977; 55:61–78.

2. McKeown T. The role of medicine: dream, mirage or nemesis? London: Nuffield Provincial Hospitals Trust, 1976.

3. Lave LB, Seskin EP. Air pollution and human health. Science. 1970; 169:723–733.

4. Farquhar JW, Maccoby N, Wood PD, et al. Community education for cardiovascular health. Lancet. 1977; 1:1192–1195.

5. Robertson LS. Behavioral research and strategies in public health: a demur. Soc Sci Med. 1975; 9:165–170.

6. Haggerty RJ. Changing lifestyles to improve health. Prev Med. 1977; 6:276–289.

7. Institutue of Medicine. A strategy for evaluating health services: contrasts in health status. Washington, D.C.: National Academy of Sciences, 2, 1973.

8. McKeown T, ed. Screening in medical care: reviewing the evidence. London: Oxford U Press, 1968.

9. Ley P, Spelman MS. Communicating with the patient. London: Staples Press, 1967.

10. Fuchs VR. The growing demand for medical care. N Engl J Med. 1968; 279:190–195.

11. Rabin D, Spector K. Factors that affect new practitioner performance in practice setting. Presented at the Physician Assistant/Nurse Practitioner Manpower Symposium, Airlie, Virginia, 1977.

12. Reinhardt UE. Physician productivity and the demand for health manpower: an economic analysis. Cambridge, Mass.: Ballinger, 1975.

13. Mechanic D. General medical practice: some comparisons between the work of primary care physicians in the United States and England and Wales. Med Care. 1972; 10:402–420.

14. Beeson BP. Some good features of the British National Health Service. J Med Educ. 1974; 49:43–49.

15. Brook RH, Williams KN. Evaluation of the New Mexico peer review system 1971–1973. Med Care. 1976; 14:Supp 1:1–122.

16. White KL, Williams TF, Greenberg BG. The ecology of medical care. N Engl J Med. 1961; 265:885–892.

17. Mechanic D. The concept of illness behavior. J Chronic Dis. 1962; 15:189–194.

18. Mechanic D. Social psychologic factors affecting the presentation of bodily complaints. N Engl J Med. 1972; 286:1132–1139.

19. Maddox GL. Some correlates of differences in self-assessment of health status among the elderly. J Gerontol. 1962; 17:180–185.

20. Palmore E, Luikart C. Health and social factors related to life satisfaction. J Health Soc. Behav. 1972; 13:68–80.

21. Townsend P. The last refuge: a survey of residential institutions and homes for the aged in England and Wales. London: Routledge and Kegan Paul, 1962.

22. National Commission for Manpower Policy. Employment impacts of health policy developments. Washington, D.C.: National Commission for Manpower Policy, 1976 (Special Report No. 11).

23. Thomas L. On the science and technology of medicine. Daedalus. 1977; 106:35–46.

24. President's Science Advisory Committee Panel. Improving health care through research and development. Washington, D.C.: Office of Science and Technology, 1972.

3

Rationing Strategies
in an Era of
Constrained Resources

PHYSICIANS AND THE GENERAL PUBLIC report that cost-control efforts are possible without impairing the quality of medical care. In recent surveys commissioned by the American Medical Assocation, 71 per cent of doctors and 86 per cent of the population interviewed agreed that "medical care costs can be reduced without reductions in the quality of care."[1] After two decades of vigorous economic expansion and technical development in medicine, with great public support, increasing proportions of the public and especially public policymakers now give more priority to other areas of national life. Between 1978 and 1984, health care dropped in public priority rankings from first to sixth, significantly trailing financial support for the elderly and education. More efforts will be made to hold within controllable limits the growth of public programs in health and tax subsidies to the private sector for expanded medical care benefits. This need is especially pressing in an atmosphere of rapid evolution of new sophisticated biomedical knowledge and technology, the aging of the population, and the growth of the physician pool and other health personnel.

The wisdom of imposing significant constraints on a dynamic industry undergoing rapid scientific and technological development is less than obvious. Despite its concern, the public continues to value highly the advancement of biomedical knowledge and technology and comprehensive entitlements for medical care coverage. But the realities of cost escalation, and its consequences for the competitive position of American business, government budgets, and other competing sectors of the economy, will require us to choose between more forceful limitations, significantly higher taxes, or increased patient cost-sharing.

The source of concern about cost relates less to aggregate expenditures and more to the tax burden of public sector programs and the public subsidies to nonprofit and proprietary health endeavors through tax abatements. When faced with competing claims on national resources, government finds it easier to restrain growth in public programs affecting the poor and disabled who constitute relatively weak constituencies than to reduce subsidies shared by large, articulate, and sophisticated segments of the larger American public. The scope and mode of financing in the health sector overall has increased the cost within public programs of meeting the needs of those with the most sickness but least personal resources. The imminent risk we face is less a deterioration in medical care overall, and more a continuing erosion of access and appropriate care for our most unfortunate populations. The poorest populations, particularly those who depend on Medicaid, are most vulnerable to loss of access and limitations on scope of services during times of economic stress. Between 1976 and 1984, the proportion of poor and near poor covered by the Medicaid program decreased from 65 to 52 per cent. New initiatives in cost containment that do not achieve balance in relation to the entire system of care will result in different and inferior levels of care for the poor in contrast to the population overall. Evidence for this trend is already apparent.[2]

Interest in competition and competitive incentives have helped health maintenance organizations, preferred provider organizations, and a variety of freestanding ambulatory facilities, such as those for surgery and emergency care. The increase in physician supply has provided opportunities for innovation and altered practice styles that would have appeared highly unlikely just a decade ago. Between 1981 and 1984, the proportion of physicians who reported that they would consider joining an HMO increased from 25 to 33 per cent.[1] Just where the changing mix of public and private, and competition and regulation, will lead remains unclear, but the dynamic quality of the industry suggests major changes and innovative future options.

Despite the evident dynamism of health services activity, attitudes are very much polarized. At one extreme are physician leaders who view the present system as fundamentally sound, who strongly support traditional fee-for-service payment schemes, and who oppose such alternatives as HMOs.[3] At the opposite pole are critics who view the delivery system as so flawed in its structure and priorities and so dominated by special interests that only major reorganization offers any promise of an equitable and effective delivery system in the future.[4] Given the range of viewpoints and interests, it is inevitable that a diversity of models will persist reflecting the vast differences among local situations and necessary compromises with powerful groups having a major stake in public policies.

There is speculation that the size and power of profit-oriented multihospital corporations will reduce the traditional influence and autonomy of physicians,[5] particularly in the context of an impending "physician excess." The aggregate numbers may appear alarming in light of physicians' potential to generate costs well beyond their own income as managers of patient care, but the growth of physician manpower also provides opportunities for hospitals and other medical care institutions to innovate in practice organization and care patterns in a way that doctors could easily resist when they were in short supply. Such physician dominance, for example, not only slowed the growth of prepaid group practice but also insured that managers of such organizations could not very forcefully intervene in how resources were being used.[6] Despite the changes noted, hospitals continue to rely on physician cooperation to maintain bed occupancy in an increasingly competitive arena for paying or insured patients and, thus, continue to satisfy physician demands for technology and other expensive, but not always essential, facilities.

Consideration of Some Workable Constraints

Under third-party insurance, and the willingness to pay providers on the basis of costs or usual and customary fees, the greater the supply of physicians, hospital beds, and ancillary capacity, the greater the number of services provided. While there are practical limits to the ability of providers to utilize excess capacity, the more the available resources the more likely they are to be used. Altering third-party insurance by increasing co-insurance and deductibles and imposing limits on types of coverage inhibits such provider-generated demand, but there is sufficient clinical uncertainty even under more stringent payment conditions to allow significant variations in medical decision-making.[7]

It is now commonplace to argue that increased competition among providers will reduce costs; unfortunately, distinctions are rarely made between unit costs and aggregate costs for populations. While increased competition among providers may set limits on what a specific service may cost, aggressive competition can generate new types of services, new demands, increased uncoupling of services, repeated hospitalizations and visits, and the use of more ancillary care. In many sectors of the economy, growth in aggregate expenditures reflect how individuals decide to invest their income at the margins. Thus, if airfares are less expensive, and more people travel, both the industry and consumers may benefit. In contrast, if competition in health care results in lower unit costs but more aggregate utilization, the results, depending on the procedures and technologies used, could be injurious to health. No one would contend that more surgery is "good" unless it is clearly linked to improved health benefits.

Few physicians consciously exploit patients or cynically manipulate the reimbursement system. Uncertainty, however, provides a context in which speciality bias, personal inclination, and economic interests are easily confused with quality care and appropriate practice. In uncertain situations, physicians are more likely to practice the skills they know and feel comfortable with, and that yield economic rewards.

Rationing: General Considerations

There are basically three approaches to constraining costs, and all in some sense are rationing devices.[8] These are: significantly increasing cost-sharing both to deter utilization and to share the burden of paying for those services that are used; formally regulating health care costs through explicit decisions on coverage, acquisition of facilities and technologies, and conditions for service provision; and establishing capitated systems that set general budgetary limits on providers but also allow professional groups to internally establish priorities and expenditure patterns. Most countries, including the United States, use some mix of all three approaches but differ significantly in how they balance them.

Although rationing is sometimes evoked by critics of change as a new impending threat and aberration, rationing of health care has always existed but has remained sufficiently embedded in common modes of thinking to attract little attention. Rationing is no more than a means of apportioning, through some method of allowance, some limited good or service. Given the complexity and generosity of the American system of care, we have successfully maintained the illusion that rationing is foreign to it.

Rationing by Cost-Sharing

When individuals paid for their own care directly out of pocket, decisions were always influenced implicitly by cost and competing economic needs. As insurance covered more costs, such considerations became less influential but persisted. Even now, few persons have insurance with full coverage for all services without deductibles, and such cost-sharing and co-insurance are significantly increasing. The Rand Health Experiment demonstrated that co-insurance has a powerful inhibitory effect on ambulatory care.[9] Persons receiving free care had expenditures about 50 per cent more than those with income-related catastrophic insurance. The degree of reduction in ambulatory demand was associated with the co-insurance rate.

While there is little evidence that increased cost-sharing associated with reduced ambulatory care adversely affects health in the aggregate, there is some evidence that the poor do less well under cost-sharing conditions.[10] In many instances, cost-sharing is likely to inhibit the poor and old more than those who are affluent, yet these are the populations with the greatest medical problems and who require the most care. Moreover, co-insurance arrangements are administratively complex and expensive to administer and ration care in a way that provides few incentives for providers to be more cost-conscious and efficient. Since co-insurance and deductibles are unpopular among consumers who value comprehensive coverage, and easily manipulated by public programs during periods of economic stress, they also contribute to instability in the system of care and uncertain patient expectations.

Despite these objections, rationing by increased co-insurance and deductibles has accelerated in recent years in both the public and private sectors. Deductibles under Medicare have been increased for both hospital and physician services, but proposals to do so further have not prevailed thus far. Most observers anticipate renewed efforts to increase cost-sharing among the elderly in light of the federal deficit and future deficits projected for the Medicare Hospital Trust Fund. Many employers in the private sector have increased cost-sharing requirements among their employees[11] and these changes seem to have resulted in greater dissatisfaction among the public about access to care and costs.[12] While cost-sharing may be a reasonable strategy for more privileged segments of our population, and are unlikely to result in decrements in care or in health status, they may have a much more profound effect on the poor and near poor.

Explicit Rationing

Cost-sharing has been creeping up in such important programs as Medicare, and in many third-party insurance programs in the private sector, but other regulatory efforts have accelerated as well. Such efforts can conceptually be differentiated in terms of the extent to which they seek to restrain costs by overall budgetary limitations without clinical intrusion or whether they more explicitly seek to regulate expenditures for varying components of care and adoption of new technologies. In the latter instance, government health agencies explicitly control the acquisition and diffusion of new technologies and procedures, specify the range of care, types of service, context of care for reimbursement, identify reimbursable providers, and even specify the frequency or minimal intervals for carrying out varying tests, procedures, and examinations. While there are many instances of each of these types of regulation already in such public programs as Medicare and Medicaid, and in private and nonprofit health insurance programs as well, such explicit limitations have most typically involved areas that were outside the conventionally defined core of covered services. Thus, limitations on service coverage are more likely to exist for mental health, dental and drug utilization, and new "experimental" procedures than for "basic" components of general medical care. Certificate of need regulations were designed to control the spread of expensive new technologies but were not applied to existing ones, nor did they much influence such acquisitions outside hospitals. In short, government has tread carefully in decision-making involving clinical authority. If costs are to be seriously controlled by explicit means, more forceful intrusion on physician autonomy and clinical work is necessary but likely to meet vigorous resistance. At its best, explicit rationing is informed by technology assessment, health services research, clinical investigation, and careful assessment of costs, benefits, and trade-offs. But it is inevitably tainted by political pressures that affect governmental action, and administrators making decisions are too often distanced from the pain, anguish, and uncertainty of serious illness and the responsibilities for its management.

Implicit Rationing

Alternatively, constraints can be applied implicitly by establishing general limits as reflected in a budget with specified levels of growth. Implicit approaches allow the transactions between institutions, health professionals, patients, and families to determine the potential payoffs and trade-offs. In theory, implicit rationing frees professional decision-making from the tyranny of fee incentives and the excesses and distortions associated with them, allowing patients' needs to define the type, intensity, and range of services to be provided, and professionals to weigh necessary trade-offs. Those advocating such budgeting approaches have argued that provision of service in such systems are determined by need and not by demand. The advantage to administrative authority is that it attains its basic purpose of setting overall constraints without involving itself in the complex details and uncertainties of clinical practice.

The obvious question is the extent to which theory fits reality and to what degree the suggested advantages of freeing clinical decision-making from fee incentives are realized. One would anticipate that administrators organizing services with fixed budgets seek to avoid providing unnecessary services, to substitute preventive and psychosocial services for medical services when appropriate and economical, and to use nonmedical professionals such as nurse practitioners, nurse midwives, nurse specialists, social workers, psychologists, and others in expanded roles wherever possible. The evidence is reasonably persuasive that capitated practices achieve economies, particularly by reducing hospital admissions and total hospital days. But performance in other areas approximates medical practice more generally.

Health Maintenance Organizations

In the case of capitated practice, we in the United States have had more experience with HMOs than any other alternative. Having grown in number and market penetration only slowly since the 1970s, more recent federal and private sector encouragement and support has resulted in accelerated expansion. Approximately 7 per cent of the population is now enrolled in HMOs, and in some areas they have become major contenders for a significant market share. The potential is illustrated by developments in Minneapolis–St. Paul, where six nonprofit plans enroll 36 per cent of the population,[13] and the extraordinary growth of HMOs as dominant providers in a short period of time in Madison, Wisconsin.

The HMO, as an organized plan to use health care resources efficiently, predates the current focus on cost containment and contemporary alarm over rising costs of medical services. As early as 1932, the Final Report of the Committee on the Costs of Medical Care observed that the organization of prepayment with group practice offered opportunities for health security at an affordable cost. In 1971, when HMOs were reintroduced as an important national health initiative, the rationale for their effectiveness was developed from the experiences of two of the largest prepaid plans: Kaiser-Permanente and the Health Insurance Plan of New York. Studies of both plans indicated that medical care could be provided at lower costs per capita without reduced quality and indeed with some evidence of improved medical results.

HMOs are a good model of implicit rationing in that once the capitation is determined, the organization can establish its own priorities; modes of service delivery; mix of professional personnel; balance of services among prevention, acute care, and chronic disease management; and many other matters. For many years, the literature indicated that prepaid group practice, particularly the large established ones such as Kaiser-Permanente, achieved considerable cost savings by reducing hospital admissions by as much as 20 to 40 per cent.[14] The cost advantages of independent practice associations (IPAs), where there are looser controls and less-clear incentives affecting physician behavior, have not been examined as thoroughly and are less evident. Increased insurance coverage, without a system of controls and incentives, will simply inflate the demand for medical care.

How do prepaid group practices reduce hospital admissions and surgical care? We can say with some assurance that it is not through greater utilization of ambulatory care. The popular notion that early ambulatory care reduces the need for more intensive care is unsubstantiated. Whenever ambulatory coverage is increased—in the absence of a system of organizational controls—utilization rises not only for ambulatory coverage but also for inpatient care.[15] The probability of hospital admission is in part a product of the number of patients who walk into a physician's office. Nor can the cost-containment advantages of prepaid group practices simply be explained by the failure to take into account social-demographic selectivity in various types of plans or utilization of health services outside of the plan. Even when such factors are taken into account, it remains evident that prepaid group practice still offers cost advantages. Selection of patients into health plans on the basis of health problems and health needs is a more complex and difficult issue, and the evidence is somewhat mixed. Overall, however, there is as much reason to believe that HMOs attract and retain persons with high health risks as there is to believe that they select as enrollees primarily healthy persons.

In the Rand Health Experiment, 1,149 persons were randomly assigned in 1976 to an established HMO, the Group Health Cooperative of Puget Sound, and an additional 733 prior enrollees were also studied.[16] The randomization process eliminates the effects of possible risk selection. Both groups studied had 40 per cent less hospital admissions than in the free fee-for-service plan, a finding that supports the aggregate literature on the cost-effectiveness of HMOs. Rand, of course, studied one established HMO, and the study did not include the over-65 age group. It is quite possible that some HMOs disproportionately attract persons with higher risks of medical need while others have healthy persons overrepresented. Moreover, the situation could vary by age group. For example, young families with children are often attracted to HMOs because of the range of services and insurance coverage that makes out-of-pocket payments for minor illnesses unnecessary. These families are often healthy and primarily use medical care for routine and inexpensive services. As HMOs more commonly enroll Medicare recipients, differential risk selection may be more problematic. One major barrier to prepaid group practice enrollment has always been the reluctance many patients have to leave an established relationship with a physician. An elderly person who has had serious health problems may have come to depend on a specific practitioner, and thus may be more reluctant to leave this physician to join a closed HMO panel.

Many studies have noted that HMOs provide more preventive services than office-based fee-for-service physicians, but Luft[14] has argued that this difference is related more to the comprehensiveness of insurance coverage characterizing HMOs than any unique aspect of its organization or incentives. In contrast, the Rand Health Experiment found that preventive visits in the HMO studied were twice as frequent in comparison to the various fee-for-service plans and even exceeded those made in the free fee-for-service plan. Most such preventive services were for well-child care and gynecologic examinations. Outpatient visits, in contrast, did not significantly differ between the HMO and the free fee-for-service plan.

HMO advocates have often maintained that cost-savings result from the incentive to keep people healthy, treat them early, and avoid subsequent need for more intensive services such as hospitalization. There has never been any significant support for this contention and all indications point to the lower hospital admission rate as a result of style of practice rather than differential morbidity.[17] Even in the ambulatory care situation, HMOs have not consistently provided more access than other insurance programs, although the HMO studied by Rand provided more outpatient visits than any but the free fee-for-service plan. For example, while those randomized into the HMO made 4.3 visits per person, those in the experimental group with 25 per cent co-insurance used 3.5 visits. There is little evidence from the experiment overall, or from other studies, that these variations in access to outpatient care have the significant impacts on health that some believe them to have.

The cost advantages of prepaid group practices seem to relate to the potential resources available to prepaid physicians in contrast to those available to other physicians and the economic, organizational, and psychological forces affecting physician behavior. Kaiser-Permanente, the plan with the best long-term record of success in maintaining a relatively low level of hospital admissions, has a much lower number of beds available per capita than the number available to doctors in comparable communities. Could it be that lower hospital admissions simply reflect the limitations on availability of hospital beds? Perhaps this is so to some degree, but it is also clear that prepaid group practice physicians, who use the same hospitals that are available to other physicians in their communities, also admit fewer patients to these hospitals.

Physicians who work in prepaid group practices, primarily on salary, do not have incentives to hospitalize a patient unnecessarily. Indeed, this may require more time, effort, and inconvenience, with no futher remuneration. Moreover, prepaid physicians are encouraged to be prudent in the use of the hospital, and in some instances are economically rewarded for conserving resources. I doubt that these economic incentives are very powerful, but the total system of incentives is not insignificant and probably contributes to conservative use of hospital care. Whether such savings result from incentives for economy in the prepaid context or because the fee-for-service system encourages excessive hospital use is unclear. The fact that there is significant "savings" associated with prepaid group practice, however, is well established.

The issue of quality of care is in many respects intangible, and conclusions are difficult to demonstrate. Variations in quality among prepaid group practices, as well as among other practice arrangements, are of greater significance than any gross comparisons between different types of practice arrangements. It appears that the well-established prepaid group practice plans that have served as a model for policy offer care that is at least comparable in quality to care more generally available.

The active use of preventive services among HMO enrollees may reflect the scope of insurance rather than any organizational ingenuity, but the fact is that enrollment in prepaid groups and high levels of preventive medical care go together. Large prepaid group plans eliminate economic barriers to ambulatory care, but they often substitute bureaucratic barriers, thus controlling the use of ambulatory services. While HMOs on the average tend to have higher ambulatory utilization than in the community at large, the similarity in utilization rates is far more striking than are the differences.[17]

Although most enrollees in prepaid group plans are satisfied with their care, many studies have reported that they are more likely to complain of delays in access, lack of amenities, and insufficient physician and staff interest. A major survey by Harris and Associates,[12] carried out in 1984, found that HMO members were more satisfied on most dimensions of service than comparable nonmembers. This may, in part, reflect the substantial increases in cost-sharing among nonmembers, influencing their responses to most satisfaction items. The extent to which reports of dissatisfaction among HMO members reflects the settings in which care is provided, or the knowledge that one is part of a group plan, or actual differences in physician behavior, is uncertain. But both patients and physicians in most studies report feeling somewhat more constrained in such settings than in more traditional ones. Since both dissatisfied patients and physicians can easily leave such plans, dissatisfaction has never been a major problem. The choice to join or remain in an HMO involves weighing its inconveniences against such benefits as wider coverage, less cost, and various advantages in obtaining care from a single organization.

One way of looking at the HMO is to view it as we do the large department store chain. The consumer generally understands that he or she gets a reasonable product for a reasonable price. He is unlikely to find the very best, and amenities may be lacking to some degree, but the consumer perceives a relatively good deal for his money. Occasionally, such a well-managed store will provide more amenities than expected, and occasional products may be better than those found at more luxurious establishments, but the usual expectation is a reliable product at a fair price.

In appraising the experience and future potential of HMOs, it is important to note that HMOs emerged within a skeptical and often hostile environment and until recently faced significant difficulties in recruiting physicians. In many communities, both the organizations and the physicians associated with them were "on trial" and were harassed by organized medicine. They, thus, followed a conservative course both to facilitate physician recruitment and to avoid controversy and adverse publicity. Past failure to innovate in many of the ideal terms suggested by advocates may say little about future potentialities in the supportive and encouraging environment that is now developing. The difficulty of recruiting physicians is no longer an acute issue and the antipathy found among many older physicians toward HMOs is less common among more recent physician cohorts.

Until now, medical services in HMOs have been dominated by a physician perspective and one that mirrored medical practice in fee-for-service practice, partly for the reasons already suggested. The little evidence that is available suggests that the physician's style of practice and use of practice modalities in HMOs reflects prior training and clinical orientations more than organizational management. In the future, the supply of physicians, and their greater willingness to work in HMOs, will allow HMO administrators more leverage in supervising physician behavior and in innovating a mix of services. Although we have not as yet seen a great deal of innovation, the potential is there. Other health practitioners will have to demonstrate, of course, that their substitution for increasingly available physician services is in fact cost-effective and that the expanded services they offer in preventive, psychosocial care and health maintenance help limit demand for other components of the health care package.

Rationing Styles: Areas of Uncertainty

The theory underlying the presumed effects of removal of fee incentives on professionals also requires scrutiny. The evidence shows that removal of such incentives decrease the motivation and work effort of physicians to some degree, allowing them to substitute more leisure for a longer workweek. This is little cause for alarm in the context of a growing supply of physicians and other health care personnel as long as these professionals remain responsive to patients. There is little evidence of difference in work orientations by type of practice, but the frequent finding that patients in HMOs feel their physicians less interested in and responsive to them than physicians in office-based, fee-for-service practice, merits some watching.[14]

In thinking about these issues for the future, the distinction between how an organization is paid and how doctors are paid is fundamental. HMOs, despite their status as capitated systems, may choose to pay physicians and other personnel in varying ways depending on the quality of their motivation and work, their responsiveness to patients, and their productivity. Capitation insures that the basic income pool is fixed; how such income in distributed to best effect is an area deserving of more attention than it has heretofore received.

In those HMOs where physician remuneration is unrelated to the number or type of procedures they perform, it is naive to expect that only medical need will now determine the allocation of effort; nor can we assume that professionals left to their own devices will have as their only priority the interests of their patients. It is human to have preferences, to pursue the interesting and novel rather than the dull and routine, and to seek activities and practices held in higher esteem by one's peers and the world at large. It does not follow that physicians, health administrators, nurses, and other professionals will allocate resources in direct relationship to need as compared with the attractiveness and sophistication of the patient, the inherent challenge and excitement of varying procedures, career needs, and personal inclinations. Patients, too, vary greatly in what they demand, their degree of acquiescence, and their skills in manipulating the system, and there is little in human experience that should lead us to believe that the transactions that result will bring comparable services or outcomes. Variability is to be expected; what must particularly be guarded against is allocation of disproportionate resources to the more affluent and sophisticated patient with less medical need but higher expectations and greater persuasiveness. This area needs careful attention, particularly as more Medicaid and Medicare recipients are enrolled in HMOs.

Experience also teaches us that equal access is a goal more easily talked about than achieved. All systems of care are under great pressure from educated and sophisticated constituencies that know what is possible and increasingly demand it. While our system of health services is sufficiently generous to soften the consequences of differential social and political pressure, it is also likely that the system will yield when persistently pushed. The groups thus at greatest risk are the sick, poor, old, and less-educated clients who know less about how to manage the system.

A budget is simply an instrument; the scope and quality of care, and the impact of rationing, depend, of course, on how it is managed. Budgets require health administrators and professionals to set priorities, and it is here that we have the least information and face the greatest uncertainty. While, in theory, professionals will carefully examine the trade-offs and constrain their colleagues within some reasonably established priorities and criteria, there is little evidence that this occurs. Administratively, it is easier to delay the initiation of a new technology, service, or unit, reduce staff and close beds, eliminate "nonessential" services, and constrain wages and other major costs. Only rarely, and at the margins, have efforts been made to significantly alter processes of care and decisions physicians typically make. Organizations and professionals must confront more directly variations in practice and cost that cannot be justified on the basis of differences in patient mix, the particular populations served, and the uncertainties of clinical efforts.[18]

The ability to ration services without divisiveness depends on the public's trust. In the United States such trust has been high but fragile because of the divisions within the health professions and the increasing visibility of such differences in the mass media. Given the public's high expectations and support for medical technology, it is inevitable that the media will give attention to rationing efforts and their economic, ethical, and human consequences. Decision-making in the spotlight is always more difficult and potentially divisive. American patients are less deferent to authority and more questioning than those in England, for example. Thus we should not anticipate comparable acquiescence to limitation of resources and withholding of services that typifies the English context.[19] The English have learned to accept many limitations in services and social amenities, and much of the older population still recognizes the improvements in access to care that followed the establishment of the National Health Service (NHS). The stable and continuing relationships most people have with a general practitioner, limited geographic mobility, and the free availability of care at the time of service, all help reinforce the authority and trust placed in the general practitioner. As Aaron and Schwartz note in respect to the unavailability of chronic dialysis to those over 55 years of age:

> For many patients with renal failure, the local physician does not even raise the possibility of dialysis. In other circumstances, however, he says that dialysis does not seem to be indicated. Because of the respect that most patients have for physicians, the doctor's recommendations are usually followed with little complaint.[19]

Another important dimension that facilitates rationing decisions, as Aaron and Schwartz note, is the stability of professional relationships within the NHS and the common interest among both general practitioners and consultants to maintain effective continuing communication. In the United States the competing interests of physicians are greater, relationships are more fragmented, and doctors are more likely to openly compete and criticize one another.

It is fair to suggest that the degree of authority and trust that characterizes the provision of medical services in England exceeds any reasonable expectations we can have about the United States. Trust is also likely to erode in England as the population becomes more sophisticated and earlier generations are replaced by later cohorts who have no memories of services in the era preceding the NHS. Trust has always been an indispensable aspect of effective doctor-patient encounters, and as physicians take on more responsibility for balancing their efforts as agent of the patient with the need to use resources in a cost-effective way, trust becomes even more essential. Indeed, one argument for rationing by external authority is that it insulates the doctor-patient relationship from the tensions of adjudicating between patient needs and demands and the budgetary constraints on the organization. Under explicit rationing, physicians can more easily explain limitations on the basis of external constraints in contrast to their own decisions and can be patient advocates without reservations.[20]

The increasing tendency to "lock" patients to health provider organizations and limit choice subtlety shifts the physician's role from agent of the patient to a bureaucratic official allocating resources among competing demands.[21] These changes create new tensions that in the absence of trust building procedures, such as mechanisms for review and resolving patient complaints, could be troublesome.[22]

The Social Content of Rationing Decisions

Capitated systems need not be based on values different from fee-for-service organizations, but they have more incentive to avoid expensive institutional care and technical services. As we provide care for larger numbers of persons who are old, we will have to rethink carefully as a society what we consider appropriate care. Medical care is only one component of the health care and functioning needs of the aging population. We have yet to face up to financing the long-term care of the elderly in a rational way. The finite resources available make it certain that we will face tough decisions on the relative value of varying types of services. Capitation lends itself to making such judgments and one alternative being examined is the social health maintenance organization (SHMO).[23] This approach attempts to overcome the fragmentation of financing and categorical services by a single system responsible for acute hospital and nursing services, ambulatory medical care, and such personal services as homemaker, home health and chore services, meals, counseling, transportation, etc. In the SHMO, the provider organization takes on all financial, programmatic, and care decision responsibility within a capitation restraint. On Lok, a successful demonstration of the concept in San Francisco, illustrates the potentialities of such an approach.[24] SHMOs have many financial uncertainties but also great potential. They build on the widespread and deep desire of most elderly to remain in their homes and communities and avoid institutional care. To be financially viable, however, enrollment must be limited to elderly eligible for institutionalization or other costly care alternatives, and not significantly opened to new populations. The dilemma is that the more attractive long-term care services become, the more eligible clients are likely to appear.

Politics and Rationing

In the English National Health Service, rationing is a product of the unavailability of resources and a more or less implicit understanding among physicians about the appropriate limits of care. There is no mandate that says that the elderly will not receive hemodialysis, but such patients are not referred and it is generally understood that they are not seen as appropriate candidates for such care. Such rationing through consensus reduces political debate over social policy issues in medical care as compared with explicit rationing by central authority, but it puts a special obligation on professionals to administer such understandings in a fair way. In the NHS, as in Western systems of national health insurance more generally, it is rare for administrators or even fellow physicians to interfere with clinical judgment.

A major symbolic value of medical care is the effort to insure all citizens equal opportunity to develop and use their capacities consistent with their aspirations. An effective system links in a value sense all classes, races, regions, and age groups. The imposition of political judgment as a substitute for professional discretion threatens not only the care process but also the symbolic value of the health care system. Some totalitarian societies structure health services to prefer strategic workers or government cadres over others. Obvious political rationing occurs in the United States as well when the Medicaid program denies payment for effective services, such as abortion, that are generally available in other health care programs. Efforts in the United States to impose criteria that arise from motives other than those concerned with quality of health and functioning could have damaging consequences for public trust and confidence. Without such trust, the system of care will inevitably deteriorate.

Rationing and Competitive Markets

However we organize future medical services, it is inevitable that public programs such as Medicare and Medicaid, and many employer sponsored programs, will have significant limits on scope of insurance. Patients will have options varying from relatively basic to more comprehensive benefits involving alternative deductible and co-insurance arrangements or additional premiums depending on the levels of coverage sought. The popularity of Medi-gap policies among the elderly attest to the desire for comprehensive services available at the point of need with limited or no out-of-pocket expenditures.

In England, supplementary private insurance markets reduce pressures for expanded or enriched services, dampen the frustrations and impatience of persons with high expectations, and also establish a competing standard of service by which the mainstream system can be appraised.[25] By expediting services for those who wish to bypass the queue, such insurance also makes a modest contribution to reducing expenditures. In the United States, in contrast, we can anticipate relatively aggressive competition for enrollees in mainstream private sector and nonprofit health insurance programs. The emergence of new organizations offering selected services for urgent care, convenience, home visits, and other supplementary needs suggests that there will also be considerable competition in care provision at the margins. It is difficult to conceive, however, given the public's expectations and the value placed on medical service that the basic care package can exclude any generally accepted medical modality. This is already apparent in the HMO sector where despite uncertain evidence of efficacy, HMOs have generally followed the pattern of community practice in use of coronary and other forms of intensive care. Even when administrators have had serious doubts about the cost-effectiveness of such units, the acceptance of them both among physicians and by the public, and the fear of malpractice litigation, has encouraged the HMO to follow the pattern of community practice.

It seems most likely that rationing will occur primarily in the area of amenities, in the intensity of diagnostic and laboratory investigation, and in the discretionary use of hospitals and surgical interventions. It is less likely, contrary to British experience, that rationing will occur by withholding or significantly slowing the use of new technologies of demonstrated effectiveness, particularly in disease areas of major visibility to the public, such as cancer and heart disease. There are significant cost-savings to be achieved in marginal areas and the course need not be too painful given the apparent willingness of the public to see the medical share of national income increase.

The trends suggest that we can expect no major transformation in the manner in which medical work is carried out or in the configuration of dominant providers. HMOs will undoubtedly capture more of the market, and profit-oriented hospitals and health care plans will play an important role, but we can anticipate a considerable mix of alternatives. We should expect more effective competition among insurance programs, greater care and judiciousness in the use of expensive procedures and technologies, and more control over marginal services and amenities. The system as a whole is more likely to evolve by muddling through and by individual groups taking advantage of new market opportunities and incentives, than by broad efforts to rationalize and reform the system.

Persistent Uncertainties

The evolutionary process in health care has the strength of avoiding major disruptions and dislocations and leaves the majority of the population with confidence that adequate access and quality of care will be available to them. A minority of the population, and that segment that is most vulnerable and most needs protection, the poor and chronically ill, are likely to face the greatest threats since these populations depend almost exclusively on government programs that the public feels ambivalent about. The elderly are an increasingly powerful lobby with widespread political support, and while we may see some changes in cost-sharing, premium structures, age of eligibility, and the like, it is difficult to anticipate that the fundamental core of the program, which is of great attractiveness to a broad population base, will be dismantled. This is in sharp contrast to the Medicaid program that has from its inception been associated with welfare and the antipathy of the population to the "undeserving poor." What is typically not appreciated is that Medicaid is substantially allocated to care for the poor elderly whose Medicare benefits are insufficient, and particularly for long-term care not covered by Medicare. With economic recession and increased fiscal pressures on many states, Medicaid programs have failed to grow in relation to need, eligibility has been increasingly restricted, and many new regulatory and reimbursement constraints have been introduced that limit services or make recipients less attractive to hospitals, physicians, and other providers. When the going gets tough, it is this population that has the least countervailing power and public support. While better use of available resources may be possible with changing concepts of providing effective long-term care, the future of this entire arena, and its potential for overwhelming the public sector, remains an issue not yet adequately confronted.

The relative strength of the elderly in the political process is suggested in an analysis by Preston, who examined federal expenditures for the elderly as compared with those for children—for example Aid to Families with Dependent Children (AFDC), Head Start, food stamps, child health, child nutrition, and aid to education. In 1984, such expenditures were six times higher for programs for the elderly, and on a per capita basis the elderly received more than 10 times the expenditures for children.[26] In contrast, between 1970 and 1982, the proportion of elderly living in poverty declined from 24 per cent to 15 per cent, while in the same period the proportion of children under 14 living in poverty increased from 16 to 23 per cent. Preston marshals impressive evidence that the welfare of children has diminished on many indicators associated with the decline of the family, the increase in single-parent households, and related poverty status, while the elderly have made impressive gains, not least of which is a 10-year increase in life expectancy, more than double that projected for 30 years hence by the Census Bureau in 1971.[27] Preston explains trends in federal expenditure patterns and cutbacks in terms of the weakness of a political constituency for the welfare of children in contrast to the growth of a powerful aging constituency.

A second uncertainty is the degree to which new conditions will change how physicians and other health providers behave. The introduction of DRGs under Medicare is simply a foot in the door; by itself it is unlikely to change fundamentally how doctors or hospitals behave. If expanded to include physician services and all payers, it will have greater impact, although ultimately cost will depend as much on the politics of pricing as on the structural system in place. While capitation tied to individuals rather than diagnostic episodes would eliminate propensities to disaggregate services, increase admissions, and engage in other bureaucratic gamesmanship, a more comprehensive DRG system would encourage competition among hospitals and health insurance plans. Budget constraints as well as the growing number of physicians and other health professionals provide significant opportunities to modify decision-making processes. More physicians will work for organizations, or under some capitated arrangement, involving changed incentives. While underservice becomes a risk with a capitated approach, Americans are sufficiently demanding and sensitive to be vigilant. The altered power relationships between insurance programs, health organizations, and physicians should make doctors somewhat more cooperative and the awareness of operating within a zero-sum budget may induce greater physician responsibility for overseeing cost-effective patterns of care.

Structural modifications do not insure changes in physicians' traditional resistance to administrative authority. Doctors are still trained to give priority to their clinical experience in making judgments of appropriate patient management. They typically are pragmatic and action-oriented, and are not particularly committed to theory, to conclusions based on aggregate data divorced from clinical experience, or to administrative authority.[28] Doctors are socialized to see themselves as responsible for the individual patient, and this, combined with the strong value of the primacy of clinical judgment, makes them resistant to administrative authority, even when medically based. Such independence makes it difficult for either administrators or other physicians to exercise control over medical work, particularly in loosely organized medical settings.

Physicians will continue to be reluctant to sanction peers, a characteristic of professionals in general. Given doctors' desires to preserve discretion for themselves, it is not surprising that significant control is difficult to achieve. It is unrealistic to anticipate that physicians will tightly control their colleagues, nor is it particularly desirable. But incentives are possible to encourage group pressures constraining behavior that cannot be justified by reasonable appeals to uncertainty or needs for discretion. One important place to start is in the area of large variations in procedures performed that cannot be explained by the morbidity of populations served or justified on the basis of improved outcomes. If physicians are unwilling to address the implications of such variations, it is inevitable that others must do so.

One of the most important uncertainties is how future public expectations evolve and how they come to affect the political process. At present, the public recognizes cost problems but expresses less concern than administrators, legislators, health experts, and industry and union executives. The public puts high value on the contributions of the doctor, wants the best available technologies, and supports research efforts on major disease problems. It wants more rather than less medical care coverage, welcomes a surplus of physicians, and values immediate and responsive access. Since the vast majority of medical care costs are paid indirectly, and not by the patient at the point of service, it is difficult for patients to see the relationship between what they pay for medical care and the possible trade-offs relative to other valued products and services. One of the most persistent findings in opinion polls is that the public supports increased coverage even if it means higher taxes. Moreover, many persons are willing to pay the price for more comprehensive coverage so that they can make care decisions for themselves and their families in a noneconomic context. System designers and consumers may have different objectives.

How public perceptions emerge in the future with changing demographic conditions and mounting long-term care costs will importantly affect the impending debate. People clearly recognize the cost pressures at an aggregate level, but they do not want constraints when they or their loved ones need care. Demand for care can be constrained by public policies that reduce tax exemptions associated with health insurance benefits or alternatively employers could reduce their contributions to health fringe benefits that presently encourage high utilization. But it is equally clear that employees do not readily give up health benefits already attained through collective bargaining, and there is strong resistance to changes in tax policy affecting health insurance. The American public, which has exceedingly high expectations of the medical care system, will not easily be persuaded that their welfare lies in a high degree of cost-sharing or in less comprehensive coverage than they have at present. The surveys, however, suggest that the public is willing to cooperate to some degree in solving the problem of cost escalation. Considerable ingenuity will be required in offering options that provide new and attractive outpatient alternatives as a trade-off for accepting plans with a gatekeeper in relation to institutional services. HMOs are presently the most attractive available alternative, but persistent marketing skill and other incentives will be necessary to enroll large segments of the population.

One evident point is that in the future medical care cannot make available all that science and technology can potentially contribute. As in every other area of our economic life, we will be faced with choices and trade-offs and these will in no way be easy or uncontroversial decisions. The process of making such decisions may be as important as the decisions themselves. Health providers and population groups are polarized in many ways, and as new knowledge and technology present us with profound ethical and economic choices on which reasonable people differ, we will need more elaborate frameworks and procedures for gathering information, hearing representative viewpoints, and achieving a resolution seen as fair and equitable. Components of such a process exist—for example, special studies, technology assessments, disinterested panels, consensus conferences, and the like—but we have to devote much thought to developing mechanisms perceived as legitimate in arriving at such difficult decisions.

It is clear that new services and technologies, once introduced, are extraordinarily difficult to withdraw if they promise any advantage at all. While many technologies may have costs beyond any expected benefits, and may be applied in highly wasteful and inappropriate ways, the fact that they have some marginal advantage in particular instances is used to justify their widespread diffusion. This would argue for better control over the diffusion of new procedures and technologies and improved processes for decision-making on reimbursable components of care. The earlier such decision-making processes are initiated, the better the chances of successful resolution without thwarting or delaying the introduction of efficacious care.

While we face a future of many uncertainties, the existing ferment also offers new opportunities. Subspecialties, profit and non-profit institutions, insurance programs, and varying professional groups are more vigorously competing for market shares than ever before. While their vigorous advocacy and sophisticated comunication and organizational skills make them formidable actors in the public arena, the sense of a newly emerging format of care for the future make these groups more innovative and more willing to bargain. The professionals, voluntary hospitals, major insurance plans, and proprietary institutions and industries will carefully look after their own interests. The public interest, however, requires that the system of alternatives that results be structured to provide access and care of comparable quality to our most needy and unfortunate groups, and particularly those that lack the influence and sophistication to insure their future prospects. There can be no higher goal than to insure that persons regardless of race, income, or origin have access to health services that provide equal opportunities for achievement of personal aspirations.

References

1. Freshnock L. Physician and public opinion on health care issues: 1984. Chicago: Survey and Opinion Research Section, Americal Medical Association, September 1984.
2. Lurie N, et al. Termination from Medi-Cal—does it affect health? N Engl J Med. 1984; 311:480–484.
3. Iglehart J. Opinion polls on health care. N Engl J Med. 1984; 310:1616–1620.
4. Sidel VW, Sidel R. A healthy state, rev ed. New York: Pantheon, 1983.
5. Starr P. The social transformation of American medicine. New York: Basic Books, 1982.
6. Freidson E. Doctoring together: a study of professional social control. New York: Elsevier, 1975.
7. Wennberg J, McPherson K, Caper P. Will payment based on diagnosis-related groups control hospital costs? N Engl J Med. 1984; 311:295–300.
8. Mechanic D. Future issues in health care: social policy and the rationing of medical services. New York: Free Press, 1979.

9. Newhouse JP, et al. Some interim results from a controlled trial of cost sharing in health insurance. N Engl J Med. 1981; 305:1501–1507.

10. Brook RH, et al. Does free care improve adults' health?: results from a randomized controlled trial. N Engl J Med. 1983; 309:1426–1434.

11. Goldsmith J. Death of a paradigm: the challenge of competition. Health Aff. 1984; 3:14.

12. Louis Harris and Associates. A report card on health maintenance organizations: 1980–1984. New York: Louis Harris and Associates, May 1985.

13. Iglehart J. The twin cities' medical marketplace. N Engl J Med. 1984; 311:343–348.

14. Luft HS. Health maintenance organizations: dimensions of performance. New York: Wiley-Interscience, 1981.

15. Lewis CE, Kegirnes HW. Controlling costs of medical care by expanding insurance coverage: study of a paradox. N Engl J Med. 1970; 282:1405–1412.

16. Manning W, et al. A controlled trial of the effect of a prepaid group practice on use of services. N Engl J Med. 1984; 310:1505–1510.

17. Mechanic D. The growth of bureaucratic medicine: an inquiry into the dynamics of patient behavior and the organization of medical care. New York: Wiley-Interscience, 1976:83–98.

18. Wennberg J, Gittelsohn A. Variations in medical care among small areas. Sci Amer. 1982; 4:120–131.

19. Aaron JH, Schwartz WB. The painful prescription: rationing health care. Washington, D.C.: Brookings Institution, 1984.

20. Fried C. Rights and health care—beyond equity and efficiency. N Engl J Med. 1975; 293:241–245.

21. Mechanic D. The transformation of health providers. Health Aff. 1984; 4:65–72.

22. Mechanic D. Ethical problems in the delivery of health services. Appendix to ethical guidelines for the delivery of health services by DHEW. Washington, D.C.: Department of Health and Human Services, 1978. (DHEW publication no. [05] 78-0011.)

23. Hamm L, Kickham T, Cutler D. Research demonstrations, and evaluations. In: Vogel R, Palmer H, eds. Long-term care: perspectives from research and demonstrations. Washington, D.C.: Department of Human Services, Health Care Financing Administration, 1982:167–253.

24. On Lok Senior Health Services. On Lok's CCODA: a cost competitive model of community-based long-term care. San Francisco: On Lok Senior Health Services, 1983.

25. Klein R. Politics of the national health service. New York: Longwood, 1983.

26. Preston SH. Children and the elderly in the U.S. Sci Amer. 1984; 251:44–49.

27. Preston SH. Children and the elderly: divergent paths for America's dependents. Demog. 1984; 21:435–457.

28. Friedson E. Profession of medicine: a study of the sociology of applied knowledge. New York: Dodd, Mead, 1970.

PART II.

The Promotion of Health, Illness Behavior, and the Management of Illness

4

Disease, Mortality, and the Promotion of Health

THERE IS BROAD CONSENSUS that the prevention of disease and mortality depends primarily on our environment, our social structure, and the patterns of behavior we adopt. Health policy, whether at the federal, state, or local level, is overwhelmingly focused on a narrow view of medical technology and intervention, and the search for biomedical understanding is directed far more to maintaining life than to promoting health. Medicine has brought many impressive achievements, and contributed immeasurably to disease management and a sense of personal security; but curative medicine, however impressive, will always contribute at the margins of health programs.

Throughout history, the idea of progress has been associated with the goal of eliminating disease, but it is an elusive objective. The prevalence of disease and the quality of health reflect broad environmental, sociocultural, and medical factors, and new risks and problems appear with changing social structures, technologies, values, and medical progress as well. Disease problems are inevitable not only because life is finite, but also because therapeutic success provides new opportunities for vulnerable persons to survive and pass their disabilities on to their offspring. The common notion, then, that successful medical care will reduce demand for it is illusory and contrary to experience.

Despite these general constraints, progress in promoting health has been impressive. In this century, longevity has increased substantially in all developed countries, and in many underdeveloped ones, in large part due to improved food production, standards of nutrition, and economic circumstances. In the first half of the century, progress was most notable in the control of infectious diseases and infant death, but in many countries dramatic changes occurred as well in chances of survival at older ages. In the United States, in recent years, age specific mortality for most causes, particularly cardiovascular disease, has been decreased, reflecting a wide range of factors associated with standards of living, medical progress, and changes in behavior. The precise contributors still remain unclear.

The history of disease reminds us of the extent to which ill health occurs within a complex ecological context relating people and their social structures to their physical environment. There are numerous examples, but one lesser-known yet excellent study of malaria in the Upper Mississippi Valley illustrates the point.[1] Prior to 1800, malaria was absent from the region, but grew to epidemic levels by 1860 with the large migrations of the early 19th century. By 1890, malaria had virtually disappeared from the region despite the fact that neither the mode of transmission, through the anopheles mosquito, nor any successful suppressive measures had yet been discovered.

Malaria followed the settlement of the Upper Mississippi Valley between 1810 and 1860 as it moved along rivers and other bodies of water that served as breeding grounds for mosquitoes. Clearing of land increased stagnant pools favorable to breeding by upsetting natural drainage systems. Railroads that moved along the river brought infected workers who helped spread the disease. During the early settlement, temporary log cabins, with few windows and no screening, allowed mosquitoes to thrive indoors, and poor living conditions and diet contributed to the populations's vulnerability.

Malaria declined with the drop in migration and increased stability of population. A more stable population developed paved streets and sewer systems, and built more permanent dwellings with more windows and better screening. All of these factors created less favorable conditions for mosquitoes. Moreover, a better-fed population was more resistant, and the introduction of cattle provided mosquitoes a more preferable host than people. In the middle of the century, with the expansion of railroads inland, away from waterways and low-lying areas subject to flooding, population expansion moved away from areas most conducive to disease spread. Within a half century malaria came and went with little input from medicine or biomedical science. Similar patterns of occurrence can be described for measles, tuberculosis, and many other infectious diseases. The point is not that medical science is irrelevant, for it obviously is not, but that the progression of disease crucially depends on the context in which it occurs.

Factors Associated with Health

Numerous factors affect the occurrence and course of disease and patterns of mortality. In each specific instance it is essential to understand the causal patterns that lead from biology, environment, or behavior to a specific disease process. But many social and environmental factors appear to have broad and nonspecific effects on a wide range of health outcomes affecting disease processes of varying etiologies and body systems. While these nonspecific effects may ultimately be explained by knowing all the specific causal processes, the more general associations have importance not only in our current understanding of patterns of disease and mortality, but also in preventive public health efforts.

Age and sex have traditionally been such influential predictors of disease and death that it is unthinkable to exclude them in any serious analysis. These, of course, are biological as well as social variables, which make it difficult to interpret effects. Women report more illness and use more medical care services than men, but they have an advantage in longevity of approximately seven years. Analysis of morbidity by sex indicates that diseases more prevalent among women are for the most part not life-threatening, while those seen more commonly in men are, particularly cardiovascular disease. The lesser vulnerability of women to cardiovascular disease is in part biological, although life-style factors probably play a significant role as well. Much of the sex differential in mortality is linked to life-style and behavioral variables such as smoking, heavy drinking, risk-taking, and violence.

Age is, of course, associated with a range of degenerative diseases and disabilities that become prevalent in middle age and increase over the life span. While medical measures can delay and help contain these disease processes, the development of chronic health problems with old age is more likely. Social policy is perhaps better directed at alternatives to promote functioning and quality of life in old age than at heroic technologies that may only add short increments of life at great financial cost and personal suffering.

In addition to age and sex, an extraordinary number of studies link particular social variables with disease and mortality.[2] While the conceptual definitions and measurements of the variables in question may vary from one study to another, and many specific studies lack necessary controls, there is much evidence that health and mortality are significantly affected by poverty, schooling, marital status, religious participation, psychological well-being, social and community integration, employment availability, and stable living conditions. These factors are more or less interrelated, and rigorous studies must separate confounded effects. Moreover, cause and effect is not clear, and the associations with health status may reflect the fact that people with particular health characteristics select themselves, or are selected, into varying social situations. Persons who are divorced, for example, may differ in a variety of ways from those who remain married, and those who participate in community affairs are different from those who are isolated. Factors connected with selection may account for some of the associations commonly found.

Poverty has long been associated with adverse health status and less favorable life expectancy.[3] Such effects are greatest for those most deprived, and they moderate after a certain income threshold is reached. Income deprivation is linked with many factors influencing health directly, such as diet, housing, availability of appropriate medical services, environmental hazards, social stress, and psychological distress. Beyond the effects of income, however, education has additional influence on health outcomes. While the schooling effect has never been fully explained, it is plausibly linked with health habits, improved coping capacities, and a stronger sense of confidence and self-esteem. Persons with more schooling are less vulnerable to disease and survive longer.

One of the most neglected, but influential, predictors of health is marital status, comparable in size to the effects of a person's sex. While marriage favors men more than women, both gain appreciably particularly relative to divorced persons. Some of the outcomes result from the alienation and distress accompanying divorce, exemplified by excessive drinking, accidents, and violence. But the marriage effect is non specific, affecting disease rates and mortality more extensively. Marriage, of course, is a powerful social institution and it not only typically provides established routines in respect to nutrition, sleep and other matters, but also involves strong expectations, personal commitments, and goals beyond one's own interests.

THE FINDINGS in respect to religious participation, psychological well-being, and social integration all probably share a common core. There is no particular reason why persons attending church should live longer than those who do not, although churchgoing is probably related to greater conventionality and thus more regularity in lifestyles. Moreover, religious participation may be associated with positive health behavior in respect to smoking, drinking, and other risks, consequences clearly apparent among Mormons, Seventh-Day Adventists, and other religious groups. Religious participation also implies a commitment, a sense of belonging, and a network of social relationships that many studies show to be important in dealing with adversities and maintaining health.

Beginning with classic investigations of the famous French sociologist Emile Durkheim, there has been an impressive cumulation of studies showing that unattached and alienated persons, estranged from the social ties and expectations of group associations, not only have a higher risk of suicide but also a variety of other adverse health outcomes. Recent studies of considerable rigor and sophistication demonstrate that intimacy and social networks not only protect against the occurrence of depression[4] and other morbid conditions, but also promote longevity.[5]

Integration into larger social networks of associations not only provides an arena for personal and social commitment, but also may offer an established and health-promoting routine, social support, and tangible assistance when needed. Group association may serve as a basis for personal gratification and self-esteem as well.

Subjective physical health status denotes not only the magnitude of tangible physical problems, but also psychological feelings. While physicians seek to identify specific disease problems, patients focus more on how they feel and how they function in their everyday activities. Thus their perceptions of health are profoundly affected by their sense of psychological well-being.

Poor health and mortality are also associated with involuntary disruptions in people's adaptations to their environment, including such events as unemployment, forced retirement, and involuntary relocations. Employment, of course, is related to economic as well as psychological factors, but for many—if not a majority—of the population, work provides a sense of meaning, participation, and involvement with others that is central to one's life. Even voluntary retirement is experienced commonly as discontinuous and stressful, and retired persons, who lack significant avocations, often deteriorate. The causal sequence is complex, since retirement is often accompanied by a significant reduction in income and change in lifestyle, and aging is associated with more health problems. Retirement, by itself, does not seem to be a risk factor if aging and prior health status are taken into acount.[6]

The significance of "meaning" affecting biological events is illustrated in an intriguing study of "death dips" prior to events of important cultural significance.[7] A death dip is the occurrence of fewer deaths than expected. Studies of various groups of famous people show that they are more likely to die following a birthday than before, and the more famous the individuals, the larger the death dip. The more famous the person, the more likely it is that his or her birthday will be publicly celebrated, or associated with tokens of respect and admiration. A death dip prior to presidential elections, and for Jewish populations prior to the Jewish Day of Atonement, have also been demonstrated. Although the biological mechanism remains undiscovered, people can postpone their deaths, an observation commonly made by clinicians working with critically ill patients. That death can be very much accelerated through psychological processes has long been recognized, dating back to Walter Cannon's discussion of voodoo death.

Finally, there is abundant historic data tracing patterns of disease and mortality following forced relocations of populations, the movement of populations from rural to urban living, and movement of elderly patients from one institution to another. While these data tend to be sketchy, they depict populations experiencing rapid social change in their surroundings as disoriented. Such periods appear to be characterized by high rates of disease and mortality until the population adjusts to its new surroundings. Elderly persons moved from one institution to another die beyond usual expectations, and so do persons losing a spouse. John Cassel, an eminent epidemiologist who devoted many years of study to such questions,[8] suggested that rapid social change undermined the adaptive capacities of populations that had evolved over long periods of time, and the effects of such changes as movement from rural to urban factory life was suggested even for the offspring of those initially affected.[9]

At a more manageable level for rigorous research, there has evolved a vast body of evidence linking life change events with the occurrence of illness.[10] An important underlying hypothesis is that major changes require adjustments that strain the biological system and result in adverse health outcomes. While the debate continues on the types of events that most dramatically affect health and the causal processes involved, the literature supports the assumption that major discontinuity in living conditions increases vulnerability to ill health.

The literature, only very briefly summarized here, suggests five general conditions that appear to be conducive to the promotion of health in populations: (1) the availability of ample material resources; (2) interpersonal networks of association and support; (3) a reasonable level of skills to cope with ordinary challenges; (4) a personal sense of commitment to some valued ideology or social group; and (5) reasonable levels of stability in living situations. These conditions, in turn, affect the individual's motivation and self-esteem and related behavioral factors that may either promote health or contribute to disease.

Intervening Factors

How broad sociocultural and community conditions affect health has been a continuing source of careful study and intelligent speculation, although the precise causal links that explain these associations are still not well understood. In some ways these sociocultural conditions affect basic biological processes including brain activity, endocrine function, and immune reactions that influence susceptibility to external disease agents and the unfolding of inborn processes.

Sociocultural conditions obviously affect how people perceive their lives and life chances, and influence not only demoralization, which may have direct biological effects,[11] but also attitudes and be- haviors detrimental to health, such as smoking, drinking, risk- taking, violence, poor diet, and neglect of preventive practices. The process is frequently self-reinforcing with demoralization affecting the quality of work, marriage, and interpersonal relations, and the deterioration of these increases the risks to health and welfare.

The intimate relationship between psychological and physical health is not particularly surprising. More intriguing is the fact that persons who view their physical and mental health as less favorable are also less likely to engage in behaviors that are protective of health, such as exercise and seat belt use, or to avoid noxious behaviors, such as smoking. While smoking, for example, may contribute to poor physical health, or follow psychological stress, and while lack of exercise may reflect less robust physical health, it is difficult to explain why persons who perceive their health as less than good are less likely to seek the protection of seat belts.

Individual health behaviors are only modestly associated, but there appears to be a general underlying attitude associated with a positive health outlook. Persons with this attitude not only have an optimistic view of their lives, and their physical and mental health, but they also practice healthy life-styles protective of their well-being. This positive attitude is not necessarily more consciously health re- lated, but appears to be associated with a satisfied stance more gen- erally.

Strategies for Health Promotion

Present knowledge suggests that we can anticipate major limitations in preventive strategies that do not take into account the extent to which behaviors we wish to promote are usually embedded in routine habits and social patterns having little explicitly to do with health. There is obvious value in promoting specific preventive strategies such as hypertension identification and control or immunization, but the more complex behavior patterns we would like to promote re- lated to eating, substance abuse, exercise, and group participation are extraordinarily difficult to change, even when the individuals in- volved are motivated. Glib assertions and exhortations on prevention or responsiblity miss the point and may even be counterproductive.

It is usually assumed that health promotion activities, unlike drugs or invasive medical procedures, are harmless, and even if the intervention strategy is unsure, at worst nothing is achieved. But to the contrary, there are risks in even the most innocent interventions and foolish interventions discredit and affect future credibility of those that are more sound. Well-intentioned interventions may harm recipients, as in the counseling program associated with the well-known Cambridge-Somerville Experiment. The experiment, initiated in 1935 by Dr. Richard Clarke Cabot, a distinguished Boston physician, attempted to test the idea that a friendly counseling relationship could deflect antisocial behavior among predelinquent boys. The study continued for 10 years with the same counselors used throughout the project period. Follow-up studies indicate that those who were randomly assigned to the intervention program, in contrast to controls, did more poorly in adult life. Other follow-up studies have had equally discouraging results, suggesting that good intentions have their costs.[12]

Even when a strong association exists with health, as in the case of a social variable, such as marital status, or a behavior pattern, such as Type A associated in a number of studies with increased risk of cardiovascular disease, it is naive to assume that public action is justified. We have limited understanding of these relationships, and the assumption, for example, that maintaining marriage is a positive goal for health maintenance cannot be supported, although such arguments have been asserted.[13] We need to know a great deal more before we can establish a reasonable intervention strategy.

It is assumed in many health education programs that fear inducement contributes to behavior change. Experimental evidence, however, suggests that knowledge and fear facilitate appropriate behavior primarily when people have accessible means to undertake the necessary preventive behavior. If they do not know how, or face significant barriers of cost, access, or personal impediments, fear inducement may lead to denial of the threat or vulnerability to it. Intervention, without good understanding of process, can be a dangerous and counterproductive activity.

THE INFERENCES drawn earlier from the aggregate findings on the relationships between sociocultural factors and health fit models of coping very nicely. Successful adaptation to one's environment depends on three basic factors: the skills necessary to manage typical problems with which one is confronted; the psychological equilibrium to cope without excessive fear, anxiety, or depression, which handicaps function; and motivation and commitment to personal and social goals. Skills depend on education, both formal and informal. Psychological equilibrium relates to social connections and supportive relations. And motivation and commitment depend on the incentives our loves ones and community provide. What reasonable suggestions can we then draw about possible strategies for health promotion?

Perhaps most important is understanding that successful health promotion cannot be based on superficial and isolated efforts to improve health behavior in one realm or another. The evidence is quite impressive that isolated efforts to change behavior, whether diet, smoking, or preventive medical care, produce short-term change, but change that rarely persists over time without reinforcement and continuing facilitation. The strongest type of facilitation is to successfully integrate desired behaviors as part of the culture of natural supportive groups. Behavioral change is more likely to occur if it is expected and socially reinforced, preferably by close personal associates, but also in the broader social context. The modest success we have achieved in limiting smoking comes in part through changing expectations concerning its acceptability in social situations and making it socially appropriate for nonsmokers to express their displeasure.

Successful coping depends in part on a sense of confidence and efficacy. The ability to implement effective behavior change appears to be linked to a general sense of confidence and self-esteem. A positive sense of self, and one's relationship to the environment, is also linked with good perceived health and better health behavior. Various models of behavior converge on the importance of a learned pattern of efficacy—perhaps best known is the helplessness model.[14] Animal models suggest as one hypothesis that individuals with a history of failure stop making efforts to cope even when they could. Other studies suggest that young people who face manageable adversities are more effective as adults than those who have been sheltered from difficult challenges. While the links between these orientations, experiences, and health outcomes are still speculative, there is a growing basis for the belief that good health and good health behaviors are linked fundamentally with good social and psychological adaptation. Behaviors routinely reinforced by the social context are more robust than those that require continued special programs.

In many instances the promotion of health is more likely to be successful through technological or regulatory means than through behavior change. If we wish to reduce accidents and deaths among teenagers—an extremely high-risk group for auto deaths—we do better by delaying the legal age for driving than by driver's education. Even the most elaborate campaigns for seat belt use achieve only modest use. Automatic safety devices, environmental controls and legal requirements frequently offer greater benefits at less cost. In practice, we typically end up with some mix of education, technology, and regulation. Whatever the issue, an aggregate strategy that calls upon a number of methods simultaneously offers the best possibilities, particularly when the noxious behavior is one that is personally and socially rewarding in some way. It is also clear that we do better to prevent noxious behaviors initially in contrast to altering them subsequently. Behavior initially adopted for social reasons or in response to peer pressures may become addictive or associated with complex behavioral repertoires that are extraordinarily difficult to alter.

Targeting high-risk groups is a sensible priority. We know too little considering the importance of behavioral factors and the magnitude of harm that results from such noxious behaviors as smoking, excessive drinking, and dangerous driving. While it is commonplace to give lip service to the role people have in their own health and the importance of health promotion, efforts to understand the causal processes affecting these behaviors or to evaluate the impact of varying strategies to prevent or change such patterns still receive little public attention. A model of health education and promotion based on sound principles of intervention offers as much potential for health maintenance as any curative medical technology. It is ironic that there is so little relationship between our aspirations and rhetoric and the willingness to support the steps to develop the necessary knowledge and programming for future efforts in health promotion.

References

1. Ackerknecht EH. Malaria in the Upper Mississippi Valley: 1760–1900. Baltimore: Johns Hopkins U Press, 1945.

2. Mechanic D. Medical sociology, 2d ed. New York: Free Press, 1978.

3. Kitagawa EM, Hauser PM. Differential mortality in the United States: a study in socioeconomic epidemiology. Cambridge, Mass.: Harvard U Press, 1973.

4. Brown GW, Harris T. Social origins of depression: a study of psychiatric disorder in women. New York: Free Press, 1978.

5. House J, et al. The association of social relationship and activities with mortality: prospective evidence from the Tecumseh community health study. Amer J Epidem. 1982:116.

6. Ekerdt D, et al. The effect of retirement on physical health. Amer J Pub Health. 1983; 73:779–783.

7. Phillips D, Feldman K. A dip in deaths before ceremonial occasions: some new relationships between social integration and mortality. Amer Soc Rev. 1973; 38:678–696.

8. Cassel J. Physical illness in response to stress. In: Levine S, Scotch NA, eds. Social stress. Chicago: Aldine, 1970:189–209.

9. Cassel J, Tyroler HA. Epidemiological studies of culture change: health status and recency of industrialization. Arch of Environ Health. 1961; 3:25–33.

10. Dohrenwend BS, Dohrenwend BP, eds. Stressful life events: their nature and effects. New York: John Wiley and Sons, 1974.

11. Frank J. Persuasion and healing, rev ed. Baltimore: Johns Hopkins U Press, 1974.

12. Robins L. Longitudinal methods in the study of normal and pathological development. In: Kisker KP, et al., eds. Psychiatrie der gegenwart, vol 1, 2d ed. Heidelberg: Springer-Verlag, 1979.

13. Lynch JJ. The broken heart: the medical consequences of loneliness. New York: Basic Books, 1977.

14. Seligman MEP. Helplessness: on depression, development and death. San Francisco: Freeman, 1975.

5

Illness Behavior

THE CONCEPT OF ILLNESS OR DISEASE refers to limited scientific models for characterizing constellations of symptoms and the conditions underlying them. The concept of *illness behavior,* in contrast, describes the ways persons respond to bodily indications and the conditions under which they come to view them as abnormal. Illness behavior thus involves the manner in which persons monitor their bodies, define and interpret their symptoms, take remedial action, and utilize various sources of help as well as the more formal health care system. It also is concerned with how people monitor and respond to symptoms and symptom change over the course of an illness and how this affects behavior, remedial actions taken, and response to treatment. The different perceptions, evaluations, and responses to illness have, at times, dramatic impact on the extent to which symptoms interfere with usual life routines, chronicity, attainment of appropriate care, and cooperation of the patient in treatment. Variables affecting illness behavior usually come into play well before any medical scrutiny and treatment.[1]

A crucial premise in the study of illness behavior is that illness, as well as illness experience, is shaped by sociocultural and socio-psychological factors irrespective of their genetic, physiological, or other biological bases. Away from the research laboratory, illness is often used to achieve a variety of social and personal objectives having little to do with biological systems or the pathogenesis of disease. The boundaries of illness and its definitions are potentially extraordinarily broad, and the illness process can be used to negotiate a range of cultural, social, and personal tensions in the home, on the job, and in the community at large.

Cultural definitions, social development, and personal needs shape the experience of illness and meanings attributed to physical factors that serve as its basis. While magnitude, severity, persistence, and character of symptoms affect and establish limits for personal and social definitions, there is considerable variability in what is perceived, how it is defined, the interventions that are considered and used, requests for support and special consideration, and illness outcomes.

Physicians and patients tend to view health status in fundamentally different ways. Physicians are trained to identify discrete illnesses to the extent possible and have no adequate measures of holistic functioning, vitality, or well-being. Patients, in contrast, tend to view health more globally and experientially. Although they may become concerned about specific symptoms, they tend to view their health in terms of an overall sense of well-being and the extent to which the symptoms they experience disrupt their ability to function or interfere in some significant fashion with their life activities. A variety of studies indicate that people's feeling states influence their sense of physical well-being.[2,3] Persons reporting poor physical health are frequently depressed, feel neglected, have low morale, suffer from alienation, and are less satisfied with life.[4] Although the causal sequence goes both ways, there seems little doubt that overall life experiences affect one's general sense of well-being and patterns of health care utilization.[5,6]

Four Approaches to Understanding Illness Behavior

There are at least four ways in which illness behavior can be viewed: as a disposition of the person; as a result of an interaction between personal and environmental factors in populations; as a response to the health care services system; or as a decision-making process.

The Study of Dispositions

The dispositional approach assumes that persons have a fairly stable orientation to respond to illness in particular ways. While some persons tend to be stoical in the face of illness, others are matter-of-fact or hypochondriacal. While some patients seek care readily for even minor symptoms, others are reluctant to seek care for even life-threatening illnesses. There is also considerable variability in people's responses from one situation to another and over time.

Most dispositional studies are efforts to understand the development of the behavior pattern. For example, most studies of illness show that women report symptoms more frequently than men do and that they use physicians and psychiatrists more frequently as well.[7] One interpretation is that women more than men develop a learned predisposition to define and respond to symptoms. Other interpretations are that there are real differences in the prevalence of disorder, that sex differences reflect the characteristics of the measures used and judgments made that involve sex biases, that women have lower thresholds to perceive symptoms, that women are more willing to acknowledge symptoms and seek care, that women have greater knowledge and interest in health matters and thus are more attentive to symptoms, and that different role responsibilities between the sexes affect the use of services. Although each of these interpretations is given from time to time, few studies successfully compare competing explanations,[8] but there are growing efforts toward the testing of competing hypotheses.[9] As noted in the introduction, a significant amount of utilization among women relates to obstetrical care and the reproductive system, and this substantially inflates the differences in use of medical care between women and men.

In any case, significant differences in responses to pain and illness between the sexes are already apparent in young children and increase with age.[10] Aggregate data on sex and use of medical care suggest that women have higher rates of utilization at all ages except during childhood, when the mother probably makes most of the decisions for both boys and girls. Lewis and his colleagues, however, have shown that sex differences in using a school health service were apparent among young children in an experimental child-initiated help-seeking system.[11] How these differences arise, how they are sustained, and how they might be modified are important issues.

The Epidemiological Survey

A typical approach to studying illness behavior is the epidemiological survey, which identifies those using or not using certain types of care or those who engage in particular health and illness practices. Other data from the survey are then used to account for these differences. Such surveys typically examine sociodemographic factors, access to medical care, distress, life-change events, social supports, coping, and attitudes toward medical care. Among factors commonly found to be associated with utilization of medical care are quality and severity of symptoms, insurance status, and barriers to care such as deductibles and co-insurance, levels of distress, social networks, sex, inclination to use medical facilities, skepticism of medical care, and faith in doctors.[12]

Patients' Perceptions and Interpretations

A third approach to illness behavior is to focus on the processes through which persons identify and evaluate symptoms, make interpretations of their causes and implications, and decide on the types of help to seek. Persons experiencing changes in their feeling states and physical functioning attempt to make sense of what is happening, and they tend to examine different intuitive hypotheses about the seriousness of their problems and the need for assistance.[13,14] A major dimension of this process is the way people evaluate the causes of a problem and its seriousness. An important function of health education is to shape such processes of evaluation and attribution so that they result in an effective pattern of care. Understanding attribution processes and the ways to modify them has many rehabilitative implications.

Much attention is now being devoted to patients' appraisals of their symptoms, the assumptions they make about causes, and how responses to medical advice are conditioned by the "naive" theories patients use to understand their bodily responses. Studies consistently demonstrate major inconsistencies between physicians' expectations and assumptions and patients' responses resulting in poor communication and difficulties in treatment. Leventhal and colleagues[14,15] find, for example, that while physicians assume that patients with hypertension cannot make judgments of their blood pressure, many patients feel confident in their abilities to assess when their blood pressure is high or low and they adjust their treatment regimens accordingly. Knowing the physician's view, they withhold communicating their assumptions or information about modifications of regimen. Understanding illness theories used by patients thus offers potential for improved communication, and more appropriate therapeutic instruction.

One of the most persistent observations in the epidemiologic literature concerns the substantial relationships among reports of physical morbidity, psychological symptoms, and self-assessments of health. In one sense these relationships may be a result of dualism in our language and conceptualizations; there is only a single body but we talk in parallel languages about it.[16] At least three central hypotheses have emerged about the relationship between physical and psychological symptoms, each correct to some degree. First, the enormity of serious physical illness causes psychological distress and perhaps some psychiatric illnesses as well among vulnerable persons. Second, it has been known for decades that major and persistent psychological stress predisposes individuals to physical illness.[17,18] While there has been active controversy as to whether these effects are specific to a limited set of diagnoses,[16] or relevant to all diagnoses and bodily systems, few seriously doubt that the "psychosomatic hypothesis" is in some sense valid. The problem consists less in the validity of the insight and more in our ability to conceptualize such relationships in a manner promoting increased understanding and improved interventions. A third hypothesis is that certain predispositions of the individual, whether shaped by biology, culture, or particular psychological histories, increase the sensitivity or vulnerability of individuals to both physical and psychological symptoms. In our current work we focus on one such predisposition: the tendency to introspect, e.g., to be particularly concerned with one's thoughts and feelings. This predisposition is shaped by both culture and social relations, and interacts with varying aspects of social situations.

Effects of Health Service Organization

A fourth approach to illness behavior is to examine how varying features of the health care system influence the responses of the patient. One crucial determinant of help-seeking among patients is the accessibility of medical care,[19] and barriers to care may develop because of location, financial requirements, bureaucratic responses to the patient, social distance between client and professional, and stigma in seeking assistance.[20] The point is that the problem can often be attacked more effectively by modifying the way agencies and professionals organize to deal with a problem than by attempting to change patient behavior. Cost-sharing requirements, distance to the site of care, waiting time, and a personal and continuing relationship with the practitioner, all may have different significance for varying population groups, and these must be understood for the effective organization of medical services.

Vocabularies of Distress

It is apparent that social learning affects the vocabularies that people use to describe their problems and complaints. It is reasonable to anticipate that persons from origins in which the expression of symptoms and a desire for help are permissible will be more likely to voice such feelings than those who are socialized in cultural settings that encourage denial of such feelings. Moreover, social groups differ in the extent to which they use and accept psychological vocabularies, and these are likely to shape the way people conceptualize and deal with their distress.[21] Kadushin found, for example, that persons who were receptive to psychotherapy were part of a loose social network of friends and supporters of psychotherapy.[22] They shared the same life-styles, liked the same music, and had in common many social and political ideas. Such networks tend to support and encourage psychological conceptualizations of problems just as certain families do. In contrast, other families and subgroups disapprove of such patterns of expression and tend to discourage them. Zborowski, for example, in describing the "Old American" family, stressed the tendency of the mother to teach the child to take pain "like a man," not to be a sissy, and not to cry.[23] Such training, he argues, does not discourage use of the doctor, but implies that such use will be based on physical needs rather than emotional concerns.

It might be anticipated that persons from subgroups that discourage the expression of psychological distress will be inhibited from showing such distress directly but will instead mask it with the presentation of more acceptable symptoms.[24] Kerckhoff and Back, in a study of diffusion among women employees of a Southern mill of an hysterical illness alleged to be caused by an unknown insect, found that the prevalence of the condition was high among women under strain who could not admit that they had a problem and who did not know how to cope with it.[25] Bart, in comparing women who entered a neurology service but who were discharged with psychiatric diagnoses with women entering a psychiatric service of the same hospital, found that they were less educated, more rural, of lower socioeconomic status, and less likely to be Jewish.[26] Of these women, 52 per cent had had a hysterectomy as compared with 21 per cent of women first seen on the psychiatric service. Bart suggests that such patients may be expressing psychological distress through physical attributions, thus exposing themselves to unnecessary medical procedures.

The vocabularies used to describe illness have great practical importance because much psychosocial distress and many psychological disorders may be perceived or defined as somatic conditions by the patient, not only resulting in unnecessary financial cost but also in increased risk from use of inappropriate and possibly dangerous diagnostic and treatment procedures. It is particularly important in primary medical care to identify somatic complaints that are related to psychosocial difficulties and to help patients better understand the source of their distress. Many studies have examined whether attention to psychosocial concerns and mental health care reduce the demand for general medical care among patients with such difficulties. The issues are complex and the processes not well understood, but there is evidence that psychosocial care is related to a reduction in both inpatient and outpatient utilization for general medical care. It is less clear that the savings that result are substantially greater than the costs of mental health services that are provided.[27,28]

Determinants of Alternative Expression Patterns

People experience many troubles and tensions that culminate in a variety of adaptations, including physical illness, psychological disorder, and a wide range of attack, escape, and risk-taking behaviors. Biology and culture are clearly major limiting factors on how such internal states are expressed. But a large proportion of what is viewed as illness in modern society appears to be the end point of a process that had a variety of alternative pathways. It is estimated that as many as 50 per cent of patients entering medical care have symptoms and complaints that do not fit the International Classification of Disease and many others are motivated in seeking care by problems and symptoms other than those they present.[29] This suggests the limitations of medical knowledge to some extent, but it also reflects the fact that going to a doctor is part of a process of illness behavior that involves such factors as felt need, perception, appraisal, definition, attribution of cause, motive, and decision-making.

To the epidemiologist, who begins with a medical definition of a case and not with the processes that lead to its social definition, there are many anomolous findings. Why, for example, are rates of depression, neurotic disturbance, demoralization, and use of prescription and over-the-counter medication relatively high among women, and alcoholism, hard drug use, and violence particularly high among men? Are these independent observations, or is there an underlying process leading to alternative pathways of expression? Why are affective expressions of depression among certain populations, such as the Chinese, uncommon but the somatic components relatively frequent? Why are rates of suicide among blacks in the United States relatively low but rates of homicide so high? Understanding such questions requires inquiries into culture, social situations, and personal predispositions.

A wide range of findings indicate that in many instances persons are unaware of the factors that influence their decisions and actions, even when questioned immediately after the event, and they often deny that such influences affected them even when those influences are identified.[30] Observations of this kind are more comprehensible if we take note of the fact that effective adaptation is often facilitated by normalization of disruptive or uncomfortable situations and maintenance of the perception of a regular flow of activities. Successful coping often requires the illusion that major changes are limited in impact and that the continuity of the person persists without major alteration.[31,32] In contrast to crisis, successful coping involves barely perceptible changes in which the response to challenge becomes part of the ordinary. To be too self-aware of change, and how one is being influenced, is itself stressful.[33]

Sociocultural Influences

The extraordinary differences among cultures in characterizations of illness, conceptions of causation, and modes of treatment are substantially documented in the anthropological literature.[34] Even in modern populations one finds an interesting blend of sophisticated scientific ideas and folk wisdom. Such cultural content affects the recognition and conceptualization of symptoms, the vocabularies for communication, modes and content of expression, and the range of remedial efforts attempted. Even limited historical study reveals how substantially expressions of distress and illness are transformed from one era to another.

The expression of illness through psychological and social vocabularies is a relatively modern phenomenon coexistent with a growth of personal self-awareness and broad self-expression. Female hysteria, for example, characterized by fainting, conversion reactions, and "kicking about" have virtually disppeared in the urban modern environment although vestiges of the disorder are still occasionally seen in isolated rural cultures that are relatively psychologically unsophisticated and repressive. One interpretation of the disappearance of hysteria is that it no longer brings a sympathetic response from the social environment and is suspect not only among physicians but among sophisticated persons more generally.[35] But while the dramatic histrionics of hysteria are rarely seen, more mundane expressions of the somatization of distress are ubiquitous and constitute a major load on the medical care system in all nations.

In any historical period the prevailing norms and ideologies encourage or constrain the selection among alternative modes of tension reduction. People facing personal troubles draw on existing sociocultural conceptions of the nature of these troubles and what one might do about them. At any point in time there may be more or less social consensus surrounding the definition of the problem, beliefs about cause, and conceptions of possible remedies. These shape how people view their troubles and what actions they contemplate.

Personal Predispositions

The variability in patient behavior in a given subculture despite similarity of symptoms also reflects major differences in psychological orientations and predispositions. At a simple level, people vary in their tolerance for discomfort; the knowledge, information, and understanding they have about the illness process; and the specific ways bodily indications affect needs and ongoing social roles. People seem to vary a great deal in their subjective response to pain and discomfort, although there appears to be much less difference in physical thresholds. Much research has demonstrated that pain has an important subjective component, and there is no clear relationship between the amount of tissue damage and the degree of discomfort reported by the patient.[36,37] What people know, believe, and think about illness, of course, affects what symptoms they think are important, what is viewed as more or less serious, and what one should do.

We are engaged at present in research on one specific predisposition—introspectiveness (a tendency to think about onself and one's motivations and feelings)—which we believe is fundamental to understanding appraisal and illness behavior.[38] Over the years there have been numerous efforts to measure personal traits that characterize individuals who display an exaggerated illness dependency. During the height of dominance of psychodynamic ideas in psychiatry, such persons were commonly characterized as "neurotic," and more recently as "worried wells," but neither concept provides an adequate conceptualization of such personal traits or the processes by which exaggerated illness patterns develop.

The concept of enduring personal traits has increasingly been called into question. There was little evidence that personal characteristics were stable across situations or over time. While the difficulty of demonstrating stability may in part be methodological,[39] current data suggest that it is more appropriate to speak of predispositions or orientations that may be operative only under certain conditions.

Introspection appears to be an important orientation in the illness behavior process. Results from research programs investigating such varied issues as self-esteem, objective self-awareness, pain response, behavior and health, private self-consciousness, and ego defense processes all support the hypothesis that attention to self increases the prevalence of reported psychological and physical symptoms and negative self-evaluations.[38]

I first made this observation more than 20 years ago, but did not fully appreciate its significance. We had asked mothers of young children to keep detailed illness diaries for themselves and other family members, requiring responses to a specific symptom inventory each day. We had some difficulty in gaining cooperation and, when we queried mothers who were reluctant, some indicated that the attention to symptoms, which completing the diary necessitated, made them feel sicker. What was so evident phenomenologically to the persons involved has now been clearly established in a variety of laboratory studies under controlled conditions.

In a variety of studies examining introspection we find that persons with such an orientation report more physical and psychological distress, are more upset by stressful life events, and use more medical, psychiatric, and other helping services.[40,41] This orientation, we believe, is conditioned by sociocultural factors and childhood socialization, and it may be triggered by particular situational events.[42]

The fact that people cope much of the time without awareness is a central point in understanding personal and social adaptation. To become aware, to become self-conscious, is an indication of more than a routine problem, a greater challenge, a break in the flow of normal activity. People can at any time be confronted with serious illness or personal tragedy. But it is not psychologically economical to worry about what one can't predict or control, and individuals maintain a sense of invulnerability by inattention to potential threat.[42,43] Too much inattention or denial distracts attention from essential information acquisition and planning, but we maintain our comfort by considerable filtering of potentially threatening information.

Persons who are more introspective probably know themselves better, and perhaps have better understanding of the influences that affect them, but they also appear more uncomfortable with themselves and their life situations. They are more prone to react to threatening situations and more likely to define many common, self-limited bodily sensations as symptoms. While introspectiveness, properly guided, may be associated with valued consequences—for example, creativity, sensitivity and empathy with others, and artistic expression—it also appears to exaggerate the experience of distress and illness.

Introspectiveness is only one of many personal inclinations or traits that may interact with perceptions of threat, coping, and the illness experience. Such traits may profoundly affect perceptions and response, the course of the illness experience, and the quality of adaptation. They may also affect the propensity to view oneself as ill, the degree of personal suffering experienced, and the degree to which common bodily signals are defined in a threatening way.

In sum, illness behavior involves a complex interaction between the quality of bodily dysfunction, the sociocultural and psychological orientations individuals bring to their situation, and the unique demands of the immediate social context. Epidemiological studies show that most people can elicit symptoms comparable to those most commonly presented in medical interactions. The challenge is to gain better understanding of the question Michael Balint[44] posed so clearly in helping general practitioners understand their patients' behavior. Why has the patient chosen this time, and this set of symptoms, to emphasize? The fact that similar, and even more serious, symptoms were evident on other occasions when no comparable behavior took place remains the core of the puzzle.

References

1. Mechanic D. Medical sociology, 2d ed. New York: Free Press, 1978.
2. Apple D. How laymen define illness. J Health Human Behav. 1960; I:219–225.
3. Baumann B. Diversities in conceptions of health and physical fitness. J Health Human Behav. 1961; 2:39–46.
4. Maddox GL. Some correlates of differences in self-assessment of health status among the elderly. J Gerontol. 1962; 17:180–185.
5. Tessler R, Mechanic D. Psychological distress and perceived health status. J Health Soc Behav. 1978; 19:254–262.
6. Tessler R, Mechanic D, Dimond M. The effect of psychological distress on physician utilization: a prospective study. J Health Soc Behav. 1976; 17:353–364.
7. Lewis CE, Lewis MA. The potential impact of sexual equality on health. N Engl J Med. 1977; 297:863–869.
8. Mechanic D. Sex, illness, illness behavior, and the use of health services. J Human Stress. 1978; 2:29–40.
9. Mechanic D, Clearly PD. Sex differences in psychological distress among married people. J Health Soc Behav. 1983; 24:111–121.
10. Mechanic D. The influence of mothers on their children's health attitudes and behavior. Pediatrics. 1964; 33:444–453.
11. Lewis CE, Lewis MA, Lorimer A, Palmer BB. Child-initiated care: a study of the determinants of the illness behavior of children. Unpublished report, Center for Health Sciences, Los Angeles: U of California, 1975.

12. Mechanic D, ed. Symptoms, illness behavior, and help-seeking. New Brunswick, N.J.: Rutgers U Press, 1982.

13. Levanthal H. Behavioral medicine: psychology in health care. In: Mechanic D, ed. Handbook of health, health care, and the health professions. New York: Free Press, 1983:709–743.

14. Levanthal H, Prohaska TR, Hirschman RS. Preventive health behavior across the life span. In: Rosen JC, Solomon LJ, eds. Prevention in health psychology. Hanover, N.H.: U Press of New England, 1985.

15. Levanthal H, Meyer D, Nerenz D. The common-sense representation of illness danger. In: Rachman S, ed. Medical psychology, 2. New York: Pergamon, 1980.

16. Graham DT. Health, disease, and the mind-body problem: linguistic parallelism. Psychosom Med. 1967; 29:52–71.

17. Dohrenwend BS, Dohrenwend BP, eds. Stressful life events: their nature and effects. New York: Wiley-Interscience, 1974.

18. Dohrenwend BS, Dohrenwend BP, eds. Stressful life events and their contexts. New Brunswick: Rutgers University Press, 1981.

19. Lewis CE, Fein R, Mechanic D. A right to health: the problem of access to primary medical care. New York: Wiley-Interscience, 1976.

20. Mechanic D. The growth of bureaucratic medicine: an inquiry into the dynamics of patient behavior and the organization of medical care. New York: Wiley-Interscience, 1976:83–98.

21. Kleinman AM. Neurasthenia and depression: a study of somatization and culture in China. Cult Med Psych 6. 1982; 2:117–190.

22. Kadushin C. Why people go to psychiatrists. New York: Atherton, 1969.

23. Zborowski M. Cultural components in response to pain. J. Soc Issues. 1952; 8:16–30.

24. Katon W, Kleinman A, Rosen G. Depression and somatization: a review. Amer J Med. 1982; Vol. 72, 1:127–135; Vol. 72, 2:241–247.

25. Kerckhoff AC, Back KW. The June bug: a study of hysterical contagion. New York: Appleton-Century-Crofts, 1968.

26. Bart PB. Social structure and vocabularies of discomfort: what happened to female hysteria? J Health Soc Behav. 1968; 9:188–193.

27. Jones KR, Vischi TR. Impact of alcohol, drug abuse, and mental health treatment of medical care utilization, a review of the research literature. Med Care Sup. 1979; Vol. 17, No. 12.

28. Jones K, ed. Report on a conference on the impact of alcohol, drug abuse, and mental health on medical care utilization, ADAMHA, 1982. (DHHS publication no. [ADM] 81–1180.)

29. White KL. Evaluation of medical education and health care. In: Lathem

W, Newberry A, eds. Community medicine: teaching, research, and health care. New York: Appleton-Century-Crofts, 1970.

30. Nisbett RN, Wilson TD. Telling more than we can know: verbal reports of mental processes. Psych Rev. 1970; 84:231–259.

31. Mechanic D. Some problems in developing a social psychology of adaptation to stress. In: McGrath JE, ed. Social and psychological factors in stress. New York: Holt, Rinehart and Winston, 1970.

32. Davis F. Passage through crisis: polio victims and their families. Indianapolis: Bobbs-Merrill, 1963.

33. Mechanic D. Students under stress: a study in the social psychology of adaptation. Madison: U of Wisconsin Press, 1978.

34. Harwood A, ed. Ethnicity and medical care. Cambridge, Mass.: Harvard U Press, 1981.

35. Veith I. Hysteria: the history of a disease. Chicago: U of Chicago Press, 1970.

36. Beecher HK. Measurement of subjective responses: quantitative effects of drugs. New York: Oxford U Press, 1959.

37. Melzack, R. The puzzle of pain: revolution in theory and treatment. New York: Basic Books, 1973.

38. Mechanic D. Adolescent health and illness behavior: hypotheses for the study of distress in youth. J Human Stress. 1983; 9:4–13.

39. Epstein S. The stability of behavior I: on predicting most of the people much of the time. J Person Soc Psych. 1979; 37:1097–1126.

40. Mechanic D. Development of psychological distress among young adults. Arch Gen Psych. 1979; 36:1233–1239.

41. Mechanic D. The experience and reporting of common physical complaints. J Health Soc Behav. 1980; 21:146–155.

42. Mechanic D. Social psychologic factors affecting the presentation of bodily complaints. N Engl J Med. 1972; 286:1132–1139.

43. Janis IL. Air war and emotional stress: psychological studies of bombing and civilian defense. New York: McGraw-Hill, 1951.

44. Balint M. The doctor, his patient and the illness. New York: International Universities Press, 1957.

6

Social Adaptation and the Management of Illness:

A Comparison of Educational and Medical Models

PHYSICIANS COME to treat illness behavior as much as illness, although they may not define the issue this way. Illness perception and response may be socially learned patterns developed early in life as a result of exposure to particular cultural styles, ethnic values, or sex-role socialization; or they may result from a person's earlier experience with illness; or they may be shaped by particular motivations, situational factors, or adaptive needs when symptoms and disability actually occur. Since the magnitude of illness and disability is a product of subjective experience and social definitions (as well as the severity and quality of the actual symptoms and physical incapacity), motivational needs and coping responses become an important aspect of the illness response pattern. Further, the evaluation of illness and disability is frequently through patients' historical accounts and appraisals of their internal experiences. Medical assessments, thus, are usually influenced as much by illness behavior as by the objective or measurable aspects of the patient's condition.

Adaptive needs interact in a variety of ways with responses to symptoms and illness. From an epidemiological standpoint, most patient-physician contacts involve symptoms and illnesses widely distributed in the population and more frequently untreated than treated.[1] Thus, the decisions of some patients to seek care while others do not, or the decision of the same patient to seek care at one point in time and not at another, are often due to contingencies having little direct relation to the symptoms themselves. A variety of studies report, for example, that persons experiencing psychological distress are more likely to seek care for comparable symptoms than those without it.[2] Such help seeking may be the result of learned willingness to seek care for psychological or psychosocial problems or due to distress triggering a sense of alarm and a need for social support. Moreover, the process of becoming ill and seeking care may be motivated as much by a desire to relieve other tensions and responsibilities as to seek care for the specific symptoms that are at issue in the medical encounter. Some empirical studies indicate that family problems, job problems, or interpersonal difficulties increase the likelihood that persons will seek care for symptoms and illnesses. They may do so primarily because illness relieves the tension of pressing social expectations and can be a legitimate way of excusing failure to meet social responsibilities. Further, perceptions of oneself as ill and seeking medical care may provide self-justification for failure when these failures pose greater symbolic threats to the person's self-esteem than the actual process of being ill or dependent.[3]

Another adaptive problem is inability to differentiate symptoms of psychological distress from those of illness itself. Many illnesses, as well as medications for them, result in feelings comparable to those characteristic of high levels of stress or psychopathology. Fatigue, restlessness, and poor appetite, for example, may result either from depression or from an acute infectious illness. When both occur concurrently, patients may attribute the effects of one to the other. Long convalescence from acute infectious disease may result from the attribution of symptoms caused by depression to the acute condition.[4] This complicates both the patient's recovery and the physician's perception and management of the illness. Although physicians may wish to circumscribe their responsibilities to the medical aspects, patients react experientially to symptoms and illness in terms of their total life situation and the extent to which their total functioning is affected.[5] They do not clearly differentiate the ''purely physical'' from the psychosocial, and the information they provide to clinicians is a product of both.

These variations in illness response are independent of the effects of stressful life events and distress on the occurrence and course of illness itself.[6] Stress, for example, may contribute directly to the incidence of specific illness,[7] or it may affect relevant behavioral patterns, including exposure to infection, nutrition, and rest.[8] Life stress thus interacts in very complex ways with illness behavior, although it is conceptually independent from it.

Illness behavior serving the patient's larger needs is in no way static; it is a dynamic response to changing personal and social conditions. It is, in part, a process through which the patient attempts to define his problem, struggle with it, and achieve some accommodation or mastery. The clinician may help guide the process by opening constructive paths for the patient, but must be careful to avoid reinforcing a maladaptive response pattern resulting from the patient's fears, distorted meanings, lack of information or incorrect information, and failure to perceive viable alternatives. In this regard, it is useful to separate and briefly describe some important dimensions of adaptive response that affect the ways people accommodate to serious and chronic conditions. These include the *search for meaning, social attribution,* and *social comparison.*

In any crisis, the people involved attempt to assess its meaning and possible consequences. Meaning is a prerequisite for devising a coping strategy because only through some formulation of what is occurring can a reasonable response be devised. Most life situations are sufficiently patterned so that the social context provides the necessary cues for arriving at comprehensible definitions of what is taking place, but for less common events, such as the occurrence of a physical disability, the person involved may have greater difficulty arriving at a definition of the experience, its implications, and the way to respond. The subjective nature of the patient's experience also often makes it difficult for the clinician to understand what the patient is experiencing, and the clinician's behavior may further alarm or isolate the patient.[9-11]

Patients with serious symptoms or disability attempt to arrive at some prognostic information concerning their problem and some indication of how they compare with others. Because the outcomes of illness and disability are often uncertain, physicians are frequently vague and evasive in response to questions. Moreover, they dislike to relay what appears to be bad news, thus often delaying the process through which patients can realistically come to terms with their conditions. Patients, however, dissatisfied with ambiguity, may continue their search for information through other patients and other physicians. Thus, they tend to obtain a great deal of conflicting information for which no one takes the responsibility of sorting and explaining. Patients experiencing a major illness or disability tend to think of their reactions to the event as relatively unique. When they join self-help groups, they are often surprised and relieved to learn how typical their internal feelings and social experiences are. They come to appreciate that their reactions may be less a product of their own failures and weaknesses than of their particular situation, and this assists in relieving some of the anxiety associated with the experience.[12] It is useful to expose patients with serious chronic disease or disability to others who have experienced and coped with comparable situations. This provides a guide to the distressing experience shared by all as well as social support and encouragement during a difficult stage in the illness process.[13]

In the process of seeking the meaning of an illness experience or injury, patients attempt to ascertain the causes contributing to their current situation. Their formulations shape the meaning of the situation, and can open or close options for actively dealing with it or the feelings it evokes. Patients may suffer particularly when they interpret their physical status as a threat to their self-worth. In such cases, they may become sensitive to criticism or rejection in a manner that interferes with a more active and open coping orientation. Such patients require continued support and reassurance that their problems do not reflect on their personal worth.

The extent to which it is useful or damaging for patients to see themselves as instrumental in determining their own condition depends on the stage of illness and its particular characteristics. Such views of ones own instrumentality are useful to the extent that they imply a sense of efficacy and personal ability to maintain control over one's life situation. Individuals with a sense of their own coping potency are more open and confident, thus setting the stage for successful adaptation; they can more readily direct situations to their own advantage than others who see their fate determined by forces beyond their control. The latter view encourages a passivity and withdrawal that may be difficult to reverse once the patient finds that such avoidance reduces anxiety. However, to the extent that individuals fail in important ways to achieve their goals and aspirations, attributing the cause of the difficulty to outside influences in contrast to one's own limitations may mitigate subjective distress at the same time that it can contribute to fresh interpersonal problems. Clinical staff can play an important role in guiding such attribution processes to minimize unnecessary anxiety and self-blame, while at the same time encouraging an active and optimistic stance that provides opportunities for successful adaptations reinforced by the patient's social situation.

Disability is as much a social definition as a physical status, and the outcome of a problem depends not only on the psychological state of the patient, but also on the ways clinical staff, family, employers, and friends react to the situation. They make it more difficult to resume ordinary social roles by their overprotectiveness, stigmatization, or social exclusion of the patient. Laura Reif,* in a study of response to coronary heart disease, found that many such patients were defined by themselves and others as disabled despite minimal biological impairment. Responses to the postcoronary patient tended to reflect the special interests of those defining the situation as much as the physical status of the patient. For example, employers excluded workers from jobs they were physically capable of holding as a result of a desire to minimize possible future economic liabilities. Similarly, physicians, in order to protect their time from excessive demands of the patient and the family, were sometimes not very aggressive in encouraging a return to work despite the fact that the patient was capable of the necessary tasks.

The manner in which a problem or disability is defined can have major impact on possibilities for coping. A dramatic example of this phenomenon is the growth of the women's movement, and particularly women's consciousness groups, which has brought about a major shift in how many women interpret the discomfort and dissatisfaction they feel. While prior to this movement many women who felt a sense of malaise and discomfort with the circumstances of their lives thought of this as a unique personal problem, the emergence of women's groups has provided new interpretations of these feelings. Many women, instead of viewing their problems as a product of their inadequacies as women, wives, and mothers, now receive support for explaining their distress as caused by existing inequalities, blocked opportunities, and exploitative role arrangements. Women unhappy with their life circumstances are increasingly able

*Reif, L. J. Cardiacs and Normals: The Social Construction of a Disability. Ph.D. dissertation. University of California, San Francisco, 1975.

to find others who support their attributions of distress to social arrangements in the family and the community rather than their own inadequacies and failures. Similar groups are emerging among the disabled, the aged, and a variety of minorities. These groups wage an attack on the social arrangements that exacerbate their physical limitations. From this perspective, it is evident that many of the social problems of the handicapped stem as much from physical and social arrangements in the community as from their own incapacities. As such social movements grow, they achieve modification of social defintions and social policies that make it easier for persons with disabilities to fulfill conventional social roles successfully. While such social action is not directly an aspect of the medical task, rehabilitation units can serve as important catalysts to bring individuals with common problems together to help identify and modify conditions in the community that hinder effective adaptation.

The way in which cause is conceptualized by both patients and clinicians can vastly affect successful coping. A dramatic example of the significance of such shifts in attribution comes from experience in military psychiatry and later in the community care of the mentally ill. As military psychiatrists learned, when stress reactions under combat were defined as a result of early developmental influences or as due to unalterable features of the soldier's personality, patients became dependent on psychiatric assistance and sought the advantages associated with the role of a disabled person.[14] These tendencies are especially exacerbated when refuge in illness brings significant secondary gains such as escape from dangerous situations, monetary advantages, or lenient reactions from authorities. When military psychiatry developed the technique of emphasizing the coping capacities of the soldier, treating his breakdown under combat as a normal reaction to stress rather than as an indication of personality aberration, it was much easier to maintain his functioning. The point is not that these patients did not have significant problems—many did have—but treatment personnel have a choice as to whether they will encourage activity and realistic coping efforts or helplessness and dependence. Much traditional medical care has encouraged excessive dependency both through the way in which disability is defined and in the failure to assist the patient to develop skills to function in a meaningful way despite the primary impairment.

The process of shaping attributions concerning the nature of illness and disability is a subtle and difficult task and requires careful monitoring of the patient over time. Although attributions can be formulated to minimize the patient's sense of personal responsibility for his failures, they must also be consistent with active coping. Moreover, the definitions must be realistic in that they receive consensual validation on the one hand and do not encourage unrealistic expectations of the patient on the other. In short, attributions must be shaped to conform to a program of graded mastery experience in which successful coping is reinforced and encourages further efforts.

Patients evaluate their skills and coping capacities through a process of social comparison. Because of the lack of objective standards to evaluate feelings, mood, and many coping responses, they look to others in comparable situations, or to experienced treatment personnel, to obtain cues as to the meaning of ongoing events and ways to respond. How a person comes to assess himself depends very much on those around him with whom comparisons are made. In many situations, feelings and self-esteem may depend as much on this comparison process as on the objective coping capacities of the individual. In rehabilitation, it is possible to guide social comparison through the informational process in a way that encourages graduated mastery of life problems. Chronically ill patients often have great faith in clinicians who assume primary responsibility for their care and who show a continuing personal interest in them. Thus, the clinician is in a powerful position to guide the comparison process through information, instruction, and social support.

A frequent failure in the care of many ill and disabled persons is the neglect of family members who, if properly informed and instructed, could have a favorable facilitative effect on the patient's rehabilitation.[15] Families often have their own problems in coping with a sick or disabled family member and may require information and assistance from the clinical team. Moreover, family members can become a very effective extension of the clinical team by providing support for active coping, encouraging conformity with medical instructions, and facilitating through joint participation those patterns of behavior most consistent with minimizing the patient's disability. This may involve modification of the physical organization of the home, the preparation of special diets, joint exercise activities, or whatever. The fact is that many family members feel excluded from the care process, have difficulty obtaining needed information, and rarely receive adequate instruction as to what they might do and how to do it.

The Use of a Coping-Adaptation Model to Improve Patient Functioning

In recent years, research and analysis on the adaptive process have shifted toward studying more comprehensively how people come to terms with stressful life demands. Not only is more attention focused on the sociocultural and psychosocial aspects of adaptation, but approaches to treatment more commonly reflect an interest in teaching adaptive skills and helping persons construct more effective social networks to assist them in managing their difficulties and insulating themselves against further strain. The emphasis, thus, has turned from ego defense to coping in a social context, and increasingly from a medical model of rehabilitation and prevention to one that can more aptly be described as educational.

Social adaptation depends on at least five types of resources that must be activated at one time or another: economic resources, abilities and skills, defensive techniques, social supports, and motivational impetus. The traditional approach that has dominated clinical medicine involves attempts to modify directly the patient's feeling state and defensive patterns, although this is probably the most difficult point of intervention. Moreover, there has been no impressive evidence that such interventions have been very effective, and particularly in the case of persons with serious impairments, it seems more productive to intervene in other ways. It is undeniable that effective adjustment partly depends on the patient's psychological response to real and symbolic threats associated with the illness, and successful adaptation requires the patient to develop psychological resources that allow the control of anxiety and facilitate continued attention to the tasks of adjustment. In all probability, however, it is more productive to attempt to achieve this indirectly than through direct psychotherapeutic intervention.

An analogous model, which I believe is instructive, comes from the field of accident research. Years of effort to diminish automobile accidents through modification of the public's attitudes achieved at best only very modest results. Thinking has, therefore, been redirected to developing technological and legal devices that achieve the same effects more efficiently. Greater effort is now devoted to such devices as seat belts, inflatable air bags, and improved highway design. Similarly, efforts other than those associated with attitude modification may be more effective techniques for limiting the consequences of disabilities and impairments.

Most obvious is the fact that economic resources lighten the load of the disabled person, diminish tangential stresses because of the ability to purchase services and create a more comfortable environment for dealing with the primary crisis.[16] Economic resources also provide alternatives for coping that otherwise might not be available. Such resources, however, are not under the control of rehabilitation programs, and thus efforts must be concentrated elsewhere.

For each illness and disability patients require specific skills and information to adjust effectively. While these may seem incidental to the major medical effort, they may be extraordinarily important to the patient. Skills may involve techniques for compensating for physical inadequacies, pacing oneself, preparing for anticipated embarrassing situations, and the like. To the extent that necessary skills can be clearly conceptualized and broken down into specific components, they can be more readily and effectively taught. Too frequently, vague advice such as "take it easy" or "avoid stress" substitutes for specific instructions that assist patients in meeting their personal and social goals. At a more theoretical level, the adequacy of any individual depends on the effectiveness of cultural preparation and the availability of problem-solving tools necessary to deal with typical problems. What may be an ordinary situation for those with skills or adequate preparation is a crisis for those who lack them.

While the problems of disease and disability extend far beyond the issue of coping skills, the absence of such skills or their erosion due to physical or psychological handicap exacerbates the patients' problems in assuming more ordinary social roles. It may be more difficult for them to find and maintain employment, establish functional interpersonal relationships, enjoy conventional living quarters, and manage their own affairs.[17] Moreover, chronic illness inevitably involves some increased dependency, and patients must learn how to deal successfully with official bureaucracies and how to manage the good intentions or curiosity of people in the community. Particularly in the case of a visible handicap, people tend to develop an oversolicitiousness and protectiveness that the patient must learn to manage firmly yet pleasantly.

A person's sense of efficacy, as well as tangible and symbolic assistance, depend on the extent and strength of social networks. Strengthening such networks or assisting their development where they do not exist may be much more effective than individual therapeutic approaches. There is growing evidence that the absence of group supports makes people vulnerable to environmental assaults and to other adversities. Often the mere knowledge that help is available, if needed, provides people with confidence to cope. During times of stress, in particular, we depend heavily on the assistance and moral support of others, and threat increases a need to affiliate.[18] We still know little, however, about what types of networks best supply support without encouraging dependency or being overprotective.

It is difficult to specify clearly the components of social support. Cobb[19] has defined it as "information leading the subject to believe that he is cared for and loved . . . , esteemed," and a member of "a network of communication and mutual obligation" (p. 300). More broadly, social support may involve nurturance, empathy, encouragement, information, material assistance, and expressions of sharedness. Social supports are responsive to the need to affiliate under stress, a need that seems to be acquired very early in life and that may have a biological basis. When levels of support are sufficiently strong, they may provide the central meaning of a person's life and thus diminish the perceived impact of almost any adversity. While support provided by professionals, or even friends, may not be able to substitute for more intimate affiliative relationships,[20] they may assist in coping with difficult transition periods in adaptations to illness and disability. When more intimate social supports exist, professionals may be more useful in providing assistance and information to those who are close to the ill and disabled than in trying to substitute more directly for these relationships.

Self-help and consciousness-raising groups, which have been emerging among persons with a wide variety of disabilities, are a constructive way of providing necessary information, encouragement, and tangible assistance; but such groups may not be effective as a continuing resource since they may give undue emphasis to the disability as the crucial part of the patient's identity. While some patients may require such support throughout their entire lives, others may be able to make successful adaptations that do not depend so heavily on sharedness with others having similar disabilities. Normalization comes, in part, when the disability becomes more peripheral and no longer the central organizing theme in the person's life. In the short run, however, such groups are a helpful basis for the patient in understanding his problem, assessing its meaning, making realistic and comforting comparisons, and receiving tangible assistance and emotional support.[21] These groups are almost always helpful during the acute phases of serious chronic problems and disabilities, particularly when they include patients who have successfully coped with the realistic problems and frustrations of the illness. A major function of establishing such groups early is to encourage patients at a time in their illness cycle when they are feeling hopeless. The dilemma is that what may be good for a patient at an early stage of illness may be threatening to one who has overcome the problems and is coping successfully. Participation of such patients may result in reliving the traumatic events of their illness or in encouraging continuing dependency on the disability-based group. There are, however, some who seem to receive great personal satisfaction in effectively assisting others to confront the problems of disability that they themselves have faced successfully. Such patients can be judiciously selected by the clinical team and given a special status in the rehabilitation unit.

Finally, successful social adaptation depends on a continuing willingness to remain engaged in everyday social activities and concerns. While withdrawal is a natural and often an effective means of temporarily reducing a sense of threat, its persistence becomes highly maladaptive. Withdrawal erodes social contacts and skills and feeds a sense of hopelessness. Continuing involvement with other people and significant tasks is an important aspect of maintaining an adequate psychological identity and one's social roles; above all, rehabilitation units must encourage all possible activities consistent with the patient's physical status. This is frequently not accomplished because clinical staff may find it easier to do things for patients than to tolerate the uncertainty as to whether they will take responsibility for themselves. A unit in which patients are kept active requires more monitoring and involvement of staff and makes their tasks considerably more difficult. Thus, staff training and supervision and the maintenance of enthusiasm are essential if the unit is to maintain the necessary activity level for patients.

The Relationship of the Social Adaptation Model to Traditional Medical Approaches

The social process of adaptation depends on the degree of fit between the skills and capacities of individuals and their relevant supporting group structures on the one hand and the types of challenges with which they are confronted on the other. To the extent that capacities and relevant social supports are fitted well to characteristic challenges, the flow of events is routine and ordinary.[22] The maintenance and development of mastery require that indivduals face demands that are somewhat taxing but not so challenging as to defeat their coping resources. The persistent confusion between illness and illness behavior, not only in the research literature but in clinical approaches to the chronic patient, tends to obfuscate the varied alternatives available to guide the patient toward a smoother adaptation to his or her illness and to the resumption of conventional social roles. It is useful to keep in mind that the medical history of the patient, even as reflected in the medical record, is far more than a clinical assessment of the patient; it is a construction from the totality of events and reactions of the individual to his life situation and reflects not only evident physical morbidity but also cultural patterns, peer pressures, self-identity, life difficulties, attitudes toward the value of medical care, and many other factors.[6]

Physicians appropriately see themselves as having a limited function in the provision of medical care. They are aware that they usually lack control over the environments of their patients and lack the capacity to change many of the life patterns noxious to health and successful adjustment. Both the lack of potency of the physician in these matters and the uncertainty of knowledge encourage a retreat to the patterns of assessment and management of the patient with which the physician is most familiar and with which he feels most secure. He treats the condition and ignores the patient, bemoaning the patient's lack of cooperativeness, irrationality, and unreliability. He provides limited information on social aspects of the illness to the patient and his family; he frequently becomes inaccessible to the patient or family who have questions and problems that do not relate directly to the patient's physical status; and he worries more about physical events than the patient's social adaptation to the community or his level of social functioning.

The fact is, however, that illness behavior and coping capacities may be far more influential in medical outcomes than many of the biological indicators on which physicians focus. While the myocardial infarction patient may be troubled by how his illness affects his job and family life, the physician may focus on minor variations in cardiac output. While the schizophrenic patient's problems in the community may be greatly exacerbated by his isolation and inactivity, the psychiatrist may engage in rituals in which he makes slight adjustments from time to time in the patient's drug regimen. The point is not that cardiac function or drug regimen is unimportant, but rather that without attention to these other matters affecting the patient's functioning and sense of well-being, treatment is relatively ineffectual.

With full awareness of the uncertainties of our knowledge in understanding the behavioral responses associated with illness, I have put emphasis on the adaptive efforts of patients and their existing social supports. In many chronic illnesses, we face situations where the basic impairment is irreversible because of lack of effective knowledge or long-term deterioration. Achieving a reasonable quality of life for such patients will depend as much on the management of their social situations and on the skills and supports they develop as on the physical care that is provided.

References

1. White KL, Williams TF, Greenberg BG. The ecology of medical care. N Engl J Med. 1961; 265:885–892.

2. Tessler R, Mechanic D, Dimond M. The effect of psychological distress on physician utilization: a prospective study. J Health Soc Behav. 1976; 17:353–364.

3. Cole S, Lejeune R. Illness and the legitimation of failure. Amer Soc Rev. 1972; 37:347–356.

4. Imboden JB, Canter A, Cluff L. Symptomatic recovery from medical disorders: influence of psychological factors. JAMA. 1961; 178:1182–1184.

5. Mechanic D. Discussion of research programs on relations between stressful life events and episodes of physical illness. In: Dohrenwend BS, Dohrenwend BP, eds. Stressful life events: their nature and effects. New York: John Wiley and Sons, 1974:87–97.

6. Mechanic D. Stress, illness, and illness behavior. J Human Stress. 1976; 2:2–6.

7. Meyer RJ, Haggerty R. Streptococcal infections in families. Pediatrics. 1962; 29:539–549.

8. Hinkle L., Jr. The effect of exposure to culture change, social change, and changes in interpersonal relationships on health. In: Dohrenwend, Dohrenwend, op cit.:9–44.

9. Davis F. Passage through crisis: polio victims and their families. Indianapolis: Bobbs-Merrill, 1963.

10. Leventhal H. The consequences of depersonalization during illness and treatment: an information processing model. In: Howard J, Strauss A, eds. Humanizing health care. New York: Wiley-Interscience, 1975:119–161.

11. Roth J. Timetables: structuring the passage of time in hospital treatment and other careers. Indianapolis: Bobbs-Merrill, 1963.

12. Weiss RS. Marital separation. New York: Basic Books, 1975.

13. Hamburg D, Artz C, Reiss E, et al. Clinical importance of emotional problems in the care of patients with burns. N Engl J Med. 1953; 248:355–359.

14. Glass AJ. Observations upon the epidemiology of mental illness in troops during warfare. In: Symposium on preventive and social psychiatry. Washington, D.C.: Walter Reed Army Institute of Research, 1958.

15. Aiken LH. Chronic illness and responsive ambulatory care. In: Mechanic D. The growth of bureaucratic medicine. New York: Wiley-Interscience, 1976:239–251.

16. Simmons RG, Klein SD, Simmons RL. The gift of life: the social and psychological impact of organ transplantation. New York: Wiley-Interscience, 1977.

17. Stein LI, Test MA, Marx AJ. Alternative to the hospital: a controlled study. Amer J Psych. 1975; 132:517–522.

18. Schachter S. The psychology of affiliation. Stanford, Calif.: Stanford U Press, 1959.

19. Cobb S. Social support as a moderator of life stress. Psychosom Med. 1976; 38:300–314.

20. Brown GW, Bhrolchain MN, Harris T. Social class and psychiatric disturbance among women in an urban population. Soc. 1975; 9:225–254.

21. Weiss RS. Transition states and other stressful situations: their nature and programs for their management. In: Caplan G, Killilea M, eds. Support systems and mutual help: a multidisciplinary exploration. New York: Grune and Stratton, 1976.

22. Mechanic D. Social structure and personal adaptation: some neglected dimensions. In: Coelho GV, Hamburg DA, Adams JE, eds. Coping and adaptation. New York: Basic Books, 1974:32–44.

PART III

The Health Professions

7

Changing Conceptions of the Physician and Public Conceptions of Medicine

SOME 25 YEARS AGO, an official of the local medical society contacted me to protest a critical remark I had made about physicians during a class I was teaching at the university. The tone of the conversation—indeed, the climate of the times—suggested that physicians were above criticism, devoted solely to the public good, and had an exclusive right to determine the character of health care delivery. The early 1960s was a period of expansion of medical technology, increased investment in medical research, and optimism about new medical breakthroughs. Criticism of the physician was relatively uncommon although there was concern with problems of access and with difficulties faced by the poor and the old in paying for medical care. Legislators and public officials primarily took their cues from physicians in designing health policy. Looking back from the present, it is difficult to grasp the degree to which the authority of the physician was unquestioned and the lack of public discussion relating to issues of patient care and medical organization.

The period following World War II was crucial for American medicine, and the choices made were to stimulate the growth of medical science and technology and not to confront the conservative

forces of medicine so entrenched in the community both profession-
ally and politically.[1,2] All could applaud the efforts toward new dis-
coveries, increased sophistication of care, and the growth of
impressive medical centers throughout the country. Although an alternative agenda was available—advocated quite persuasively by the
Committee on the Costs of Medical Care that carried out detailed
studies in the 1920s and anticipated the current medical care debate
by many decades[3]—there was little inclination on the part of government, professionals, or politicians to confront the forces of organized medicine. Everyone could applaud the pursuit of Nobel
prizes.

New knowledge and technology made significant contributions,
but the investment we made in the decades following World War II
also exacerbated the problems we now face, such as an inability to
control costs and too many subspecialists. Moreover, new knowledge
and technology have brought other problems as well, tempering to
some degree our expectations of the extent to which technology itself
can solve deep human problems.

While the public applauded the growing technical sophistication
of medicine and supported more medical research and new and more
sophisticated hospitals, they did not and perhaps still do not appreciate the link between the benefits they value and associated costs.
As medicine promised more of value, the public demanded more
care; and the growth of third-party insurance and government programs increasingly shielded the population from what they were actually paying. If access was difficult, the diagnosis was that we
needed more doctors; and thus both the Congress and state legisla-
tures accelerated investments in new medical schools and expanded
enrollment in existing ones. All of these trends—increased knowledge and technology and subspecialization, the growth of third-party
payment, rising public expectations, and more doctors—are the
foundation of the current cost crisis.

With Medicare and Medicaid, and other important federal health
programs, government became intimately involved in regulating
health care and developing incentives for modifying organizational
arrangements.[4] Medicine up to the 1960s maintained a united front
in public despite internal cleavages between town and gown, among
specialities, and between institutional and community care. The
availability of public monies, however, brought these strains into the
open and doctors began publicly debating—and sometimes debas-

ing—one another. While in prior decades malpractice litigation was made near impossible by the difficulty of locating physicians to testify against one another, physicians were now more likely to criticize each other in court and elsewhere. In short, there was no longer one voice speaking for medicine.

Social change also brought more challenge to the professional dominance of medicine relative to other health occupations.[5] In the 1960s and 1970s, there were massive increases in professional and technical manpower in health, and these groups increasingly organized and unionized. Nurses fought more aggressively not only for improved wages and fringe benefits, but also for more autonomy from physicians. Psychologists escaped the dominance of psychiatrists over the services they could provide, and began to establish an independent domain. House staff began to bargain collectively, insisting that they be paid commensurately with the services they offered, and brought issues of quality of service, staffing, equipment provision, and related issues to the bargaining table. Hospital employees further eroded physician control through the provisions of contracts won through collective bargaining, creating pressure for more centralized administrative control. And court rulings in a variety of malpractice and other cases made it clear that hospitals were responsible for staff actions, building further incentives for administrative centralization. As the organizational structures of medical practice became more varied, physicians frequently had conflicting interests among themselves and with other health providers that would surface in the public arena.

The 1960s were also years of great cultural turmoil. The Vietnam War and its aftermath contributed to an erosion of faith in government and serious questioning about the uses and misuses of technology and science. The Vietnam era resulted in an attack not only upon the military establishment and national policymakers, but on authority and professional expertise more widely, and trust in all social institutions suffered.

While on the surface social protest was demonstrating the vulnerability of leadership, deeper ethical and social dilemmas were becoming more evident, and they were often issues that required long term solutions and, thus, considerable trust in leaders. The optimistic beliefs in scientific and technological progress, and in the creative exploitation of natural resources, were increasingly confronting new concerns—questions about population density, depletion of natural resources, pollution and environmental causes of disease, the ethical implications of prolonging life, and the destructive consequences of rapid technological development on culture, on a sense of community, and on the physical environment. While the optimism of the 1960s suggested that we could solve all problems if we had the resolve, the present view is that we have little facility in solving any.

Many youngsters of the '60s are now the new lawyers, doctors, and professors of the '80s. Although they have changed with age and with the times, the legacy of their socialization remains and has contributed to certain transformations in the social arenas they inhabit. While many remain socially and politically conservative, they constitute a more heterogeneous population in values, in political and social viewpoints, and in receptivity to innovative organizational forms and patterns of health care delivery. There is clearly a significant generation gap between many younger and older health professionals.

The growth of the health sector, its economic importance, and the large fiscal and regulatory responsibility of government have focused the interest not only of bureaucrats, but also the mass media and the general public. A large corps of writers and critics report on, research, and analyze the system from every aspect, creating a small-scale industry whose results get increasing attention in the daily press. The average person appears to have developed a split image of medicine: the first gleaned from their personal experiences and those of their relatives; the second a more abstract view reflecting social commentary. Both aspects of the image require examination.

Two-thirds of the public now believe that people are beginning to lose faith in doctors.[6] Ironically, the growth of public disillusionment with physicians as a professional group has accompanied magnificant advances in biomedical knowledge and technology, dramatic improvements in longevity, and impressive increases in access to medical care despite some continuing inadequacies. In some sense, Aaron Wildavsky's catchy phrase of "Doing Better but Feeling Worse"[7] characterizes the situation.

While survey evidence on perceptions of physicians indicate a significant erosion of esteem in general, the vast majority of patients continue to view their personal physician as having many of the commendable attributes perceived as absent in the profession at large. This discrepancy between the public image and the view of one's own physician has been known for some time, but changes in both the complexity of medical care and how it is practiced are likely to create new strains in the future that may bring the personal view closer to the public image.

The abstract view of medicine and medical care is shaped by public discussion as reflected in television, movies, newspapers, and magazines. It is reasonably clear that the monolithic public image of doctors selflessly dedicated to the individual welfare of their patients has been replaced by a more heterogeneous set of images. This more complex view reflects in part the increased education and growing sophistication of the public and its skepticism of the technical expert. It also reflects the fact that, unlike in the past, the public is audience to the internal divisions among physicians and medical experts and their testimony about the fads and foibles of health care practice. Unlike earlier eras, the public now has at least some conception of the uses and abuses of new technologies, the prevalence of medical malpractice, and the dilemma of rising and uncontrollable medical care costs.

It should not be surprising that the image of doctors in general is shaped by the salient public issues and debates on the organization of medical care. Patient's personal needs and experiences are not unimportant, but many of these images are dissociated from personal experience or relate to areas where the patient has no personal basis for judgment. Public concern in previous decades centered on such issues as inadequate access to medical care, the growth of medical specialization, and the perception of a physician shortage, particularly in relation to rural areas and the poor; the current focus derives from the intense attention now devoted to medical care costs in government forums and in the media. Approximately two-thirds of the population now feel that doctors are too interested in money. They also commonly assert that physicians' fees are unreasonable, and that doctors are making little effort to hold costs down.

The public sees physicians as major culprits in exacerbating cost problems. A majority believe that "most doctors charge more than they are worth," and almost three-quarters believe doctors and hospitals charge more because they know people are covered by health insurance. A majority believe that the large profits made by doctors and hospitals account for increasing costs. Also, the public is more willing to have government regulate and control physician fees and hospital costs than professionals would like.

The difference in perceptions of medical care problems by physicians and the public is potentially an explosive issue. Neither the public nor physicians appear to have a balanced analytic view of the nature of the cost problem, although both groups recognize it as the major problem facing medicine. Physicians, for the most part, support approaches to cost and organizational issues that modify to the least extent possible their usual way of doing business. They continue strong advocacy of private insurance, fee-for-service practice, and usual and customary fees, and oppose capitation and government regulation. While patients tend to blame doctors for cost problems, doctors are more likely to see the source of the problem in unnecessary utilization, trivial complaints, and excessively demanding patients.

The public view also embodies significant contradictions. While alarmed by cost, patients continue to actively support the search for new biomedical knowledge and new technology, and desire comprehensive insurance programs that protect not only against high cost incidents of illness but also smaller out-of-pocket expenditures. The type of insurance the public values, however, eliminates all barriers to utilization and significantly encourages cost escalation. While people understand this, they also believe that when seriously ill they should have the best that biomedical knowledge and technology permits. They also hold high, and often unrealistic, expectations of what the physician and new technologies can achieve. Being firm believers in biomedical progress, they commonly seek a "biomedical fix" for intractable problems associated with the effects of established lifestyles, environmental risks, and poorly understood disease processes. The profession has contributed to these unrealistic expectations by self-promotion, exaggeration, and poor educational efforts, but our escalating rhetoric is also a more general manifestation of our optimism, our politics, and the way the mass media handles scientific claims.

The picture that emerges of public perceptions is considerably different when questions focus on respondents' experiences with their personal physician and in respect to their most recent personal encounters. Patients typically assume the technical competence of physicians but seek warmth and interest in them as individuals, particularly in the face of frightening or debilitating illness. Interest is assessed by the doctor providing the patient enough time, encouraging the patient to ask questions, providing appropriate feedback, and the like. A simple gesture, such as calling a patient in the midst of a serious illness episode to ask how they are doing, often makes a dramatic impression and affects how the patient comes to regard the physician.

Most patients feel that at least their personal physician must meet these expectations. Most report that their personal doctors spend enough time with them and explain things well, but they have a very different conception of physicians in general. In part, the favorable specific view may reflect the patient's needs to trust and believe in their doctor and the fact that their current physician may have been selected to be compatible with their needs and tastes. Patients, in contrast, may have less control over physicians to whom they are referred for consultation or who provide care to them during hospitalization. The available studies do not probe sufficiently deeply to explain the contradictions and ambivalence.

Superficial images also do not capture the deep and ambivalent feelings patients have about illness, dependency, and their relationships with physicians. While on the one hand they may have very high and unrealistic expectations of what the doctor should do for them, on the other they resent their feelings of dependency. Many patients appear to want parental-type authority in their doctors but, like adolescents, feel rebellious as well. Even small and inadvertent cues suggesting disinterest or distraction can elicit deep negative feelings.

Dissatisfaction is more readily elicited among chronically ill or impaired patients and their families who are frustrated in part by intractable problems and in part by difficulties in obtaining feedback and advice that works. Such difficulties are inherent in the uncertainties and complexities of the clinical situation as much as in failures of medical care, although physicians can often do more than they do to provide information or promote functioning. In a moving article, Dr. DeWitt Stetten, a distinguished physician and medical administrator, discussed his frustrations in coping with macular degeneration, a condition resulting in blindness. He notes: "Through all of these years, and despite many contacts with skilled and experienced professionals, no opthamologist has at any time suggested any devices that might be of assistance to me. No opthamologist has mentioned any of the many ways in which I could stem the deterioration in the quality of my life."[8] These observations about opthamology could be applied to almost any other specialty.

Some patients are resentful because they believe they suffered from physician error and insensitivity to their needs. While most patients report personal satisfaction, the growing negative images probably reflect in some measure the neglect of caring in patient transactions, the hurried pace and schedule of many physicians, and problems resulting from poor communication among doctors and other health professionals managing the patient's care in complex illness situations.

Although physicians feel they know what is in the public's interest on the basis of their training and clinical experience, it has been amply demonstrated that the best predictor of physicians' responses to organizational innovations and changes is their political identification and personal self-interest.[9,10] Patients have a large reservoir of good will toward doctors, but it will erode if physicians fail to be more adaptive. Physicians' preference for fee-for-service practice in the United States arises more because they are used to it and feel comfortable with it than for any other reason. Cross-national experience demonstrates that physicians support whatever system of remuneration they are accustomed to as long as they perceive the existing system as fair.[11]

Existing trends suggest that fragmentation among doctors will increase and perhaps lead to greater acrimony within the profession. Certainly the extreme right and left wings of medicine are more polarized than ever before, and the American Medical Association has increasing difficulty in formulating policies that hold its membership together. In addition, the profession is deeply divided on many important health policy issues and a majority hold their view strongly, making compromise more difficult. There are major differences between young and old physicians, between office-based and organizationally based doctors, and between general practitioners and surgeons as compared with other types of specialists, such as pediatricians, psychiatrists, and internists.[12] Women in medicine tend to have less traditional views, and the proportions of women among younger doctors is increasing. Moreover, with more doctors and heavier competition, medicine is destined to have greater difficulty in keeping its political house in order.

Physicians feel besieged by new demands resulting from government regulation, court decisions, economic restraints, and growing ethical concerns that arise from a changing social milieu, the adoption of new lifesaving technologies, and rapidly increasing knowledge. Not only are the dilemmas in decision-making more complicated than ever before—decisions about extending life, providing heroic care, measuring large risks and costs against possible benefits—but they also take place in a context of monitoring, regulation, and public scrutiny. It is not too difficult to understand why physicians feel uneasy and stressed, why many cope by restricting their efforts to small areas of expertise in which they feel they can master and control their work, and why they feel concerned about growing intrusions on their autonomy.

One typical way physicians deal with their own uncertainty and anxiety about errors is to project an image of authority. But sophisticated consumers are critical of such behavior, viewing it as insensitive and arrogant, and paternalism in doctor-patient relationships is itself under attack. Patients are demanding new types of relationships in which they share in decision-making. Obstetricians have perhaps felt these pressures more than other specialists, but a better-educated public is imposing new expectations. As the media cover medical developments more closely, patients may be better informed than their physicians on particular options for treatment, and the courts are demanding from physicians a higher level of informed consent in treatment and greater responsibility to inform patients of risks and alternative available treatments.

The public has developed increasingly complex expectations of physicians, demands that are almost impossible to meet. Doctors are expected to be technically proficient and to keep up with rapidly changing knowledge. They are to be warm, compassionate, responsive, and personally concerned. They should be sophisticated not only about narrow medical concerns but also about such varied areas as psychiatric illness, alcoholism, sexuality, the management of chronic disease, and the appropriate handling of death. They should be involved in peer review and quality of care efforts and be sensitive to informed consent and other ethical issues. But they also should be productive, pursue cost-effective practice, and have a broad picture of social as well as medical needs. Even the very best can stagger under this load—perhaps it is the most conscientious who do.

Given the demands of physicians, it seems that they will best be able to cope in organizational settings that can appropriately link their work with the efforts of other professionals, paraprofessionals, and administrative and managerial personnel, and that provide the tools necessary for effective practice beyond the economic or informational capacity of a single-handed or small practice. Younger doctors realize this and increasingly choose group settings, but older physicians—more set in their ways—find it difficult to make the accommodations to others that are necessary in a group setting. It seems clear, however, that practice in organizations is the wave of the future, and both doctors and patients increasingly will have to work out appropriate relationships in such contexts.

With cost pressures, government at every level is intimately involved in almost every aspect of medical planning and medical care, including capital investment, pricing, and new technologies. Increased decision-making authority has also been shifted from the profession to private corporations and the courts. It is evident that we are living simultaneously in an era of rationing and commercialization, however we characterize it. Until recently, medicine usually ranked first in the public's priorities; people are now more inclined to feel that we are spending too little on education, financial support for the needy and the elderly, the environment, and retraining the unemployed. And at the operational level, the perceptions of the need for limits on health expenditures are reflected in support for such varied initiatives as rate regulation, DRGs, and preferred provider organizations (PPOs) among other mechanisms.

If the public image of medicine is to remain high, the framework for allocation of health resources must be equitable and doctors and patients must relate to one another in a trusting way. While many of the opportunities and constraints in the future will not be under the sole or even primary control of the profession, there is much that the profession can do to reassure the public that the profession acts primarily in the public interest. The population is not foolish, and accepts realistic pursuit of self-interest on the part of physicians if it remains within reasonable bounds. But when two-thirds of the population believes that doctors are too interested in making money, and more than a quarter describe their personal doctor in that way,[6] there is some suggestion that the bounds have been exceeded.

If physicians are to retain public confidence, they must not only take responsibility for providing good care to their own patients but also for the profession of medicine as a whole. The profession must develop and encourage incentives for the types of care that the profession believes needs emphasis and reduce unnecessary procedures. While such efforts naturally bring out divisions among medical sectors and specialties, these questions must be addressed. If doctors fail to reexamine the balance between cognitive and technical skills, ambulatory and inpatient care, or hospital and home care, others will.

Physicians, employed in growing numbers by major corporations, HMOs, and proprietary enterprises, will be pressured to yield some of their traditional autonomy and authority to administrators whose task it is to insure a margin of profit or at least solvency under more competitive conditions. The extent of intrusion into the doctor's traditional clinical responsiblities will depend on how effectively physicians as peers can arrive at reasonable standards of care, communicate them effectively, control those who consistently deviate, and assume responsibility as a group for protecting the financial viability of the newly emerging "medical firms."

There are those both within and outside medicine who are skeptical that physicians will cooperate sufficiently in these collective endeavors or that the behavior change necessary to avoid administrative intrusions will occur. The general public, I believe, continues to have confidence in doctors and would welcome evidence that the profession is addressing these important issues. The public is the physician's strongest ally in resisting excessive intrusion of private and public administrative authority. But the public must believe that physicians are making necessary efforts to deal with waste and abuse. The growing supply of physicians and the realities of an emerging public consensus among employers, government, and much of the educated public about the need to control costs suggest that public pressures and the threat of administrative interventions will introduce stronger inducements for physician self-regulation than ever before.

We underestimate the deterrent value of feedback, and making physicians aware that their practice patterns depart markedly from peers. Well-organized comparative information, appropriately combined with carefully structured standards that peers arrive at, contributes to restraining questionable practices. More important, such efforts can encourage physicians into a different frame of mind involving more thought to the incremental value of procedures and services. Economic incentives inherent in current payment mechanisms are very powerful, but it is cynical to assume that physicians respond only to financial incentives and in any case, these incentives are changing. There will remain persistent individualists or those so alienated from their fellows to be relatively immune to peer opinion, however effectively organized. The ample supply of physicians and the countervailing threat implied, however, should make it possible to exercise more effective peer review than in the past.

Doctors have typically been ingenious in responding to reimbursement incentives and in measuring clinical productivity. Comparable thought, however, has not been given to incentives within non-fee-for-service practice. With larger integrated systems of care, there will be much to learn about measuring and rewarding merit, however conceptualized, from other organizations typically employing professionals.

Higher education offers an instructive analogy in that the professoriat makes many of the same claims as physicians for professional responsibility and task autonomy. Professors, like doctors, have traditionally maintained that only their peers can judge them appropriately, and while they may grudgingly acknowledge the power of administration if not its moral authority, only some would acknowledge that the ordinary student can make an informed appraisal of even their teaching capacities. Yet in recent years, universities have monitored in more complex ways not only faculty work load and research productivity but also teaching effectiveness as measured by student response as well as peer assessment. Most observers believe that this improves performance. Such data now play a larger role in evaluations of performance and awarding merit pay, special recognition, paid research leave, funds for supportive services and equipment, and promotions.

Groups of physicians, I suggest, could readily use improved data as a basis for encouraging and rewarding merit. Such information might include not only usual productivity and reputational criteria but also the results of record audits, data from simple sample monitoring of patient satisfaction following physician encounters, and evidence of cooperativeness in achieving necessary group objectives. As payment of physicians shifts from fee-for-service to alternative arrangements we can anticipate some unwanted adjustments. Salaried physicians, in contrast to those on fee-for-service, typically work fewer hours and some would contend less hard as well, and patients in HMOs in contrast to fee-for-service practice more often report less physician interest in them. Physicians have not as yet demonstrated their usual ingenuity in devising incentives within salaried practice that encourage desired performance. The key point is that how the community pays for medical care and how doctors are paid are separable issues. The debate about the former issue has obscured possibilities for devising innovative payment approaches and other forms of recognition.

I suspect that many physicians do not welcome more stringent regulation from peers and even more strongly will resist the suggestion that patient responses to clinical encounters ought to be given more credence. While the value of sample auditing of encounters should not be exaggerated, if approached sensibly it could have a number of beneficial effects. Most important, the results of monitoring are instructive for typical physicians wanting to improve their practices, and the approach itself encourages self-awareness and the need for improved communication.

Changes in financing will tilt the physician's role from advocate of the individual patient toward a role with greater responsibilities for allocation of fixed budgets. These changes inevitably bring challenges to trust, and possibilities for increased conflict with some patients. If trust is to remain strong, doctors will have to be proficient as communicators and educators, and will need not only empathy but a willingness to share more information with patients. Physician groups communicating their interest in what their patients think, and who provide ready opportunities for feedback and resolution of misunderstandings and grievances, can do much to sustain trust under rapidly changing conditions.

Current initiatives encourage locking patients into provider organizations that take full responsibility for the patient's care. The constraint on choice as in prepaid group practice and preferred provider organizations may be necessary in light of other goals, but it also puts a special burden on these plans to facilitate careful matching of patient and doctor, encourage choice to the extent possible, allow patients to readily change doctors, and insure simple and informal ways for dealing expeditiously with patient complaints. The constraint on choice subtly affects doctor-patient communication and maintenance of trust, particularly under stress. Trust-building efforts will be increasingly essential.

The future for physicians, with more competitors and tough economic constraints, may not seem as inviting as the past. But neither the public nor physicians should lose sight of the magnificent achievements of recent decades or the future potential of biomedical and social innovation. The American public will continue to support a generous medical care system. But physicians, too, must see the urgency of their responsibilities clearly and the need to reassure patients that private interests will not displace their essential obligations to patients. Constraints are inevitable, but governmental or corporate authority over the medical care system is not. It remains to be seen whether the profession can regain the initiative and the degree to which the future framework for patient care will be established by external forces.

References

1. Mechanic D. Social changes affecting medical training and practice. In: Coombs RH, Vincent CE, eds. Psychosocial aspects of medical training. Springfield, Ill.: Charles C. Thomas, 1971:525–546.

2. Richmond J. Currents in American medicine. Cambridge, Mass.: Harvard U Press, 1969.

3. Committee on Costs of Medical Care. Medical care for the American people. Washington, D.C.: Public Health Service, 1970.

4. Lewis C, Fein R, Mechanic D. A right to health: the problem of access to primary medical care. New York: Wiley-Interscience, 1976.

5. Freidson E. Professional dominance: the social structure of medical care. Chicago: Aldine, 1970.

6. American Medical Association. Physician opinion on health care issues: 1984. Chicago: American Medical Association, September 1984.

7. Wildavsky A. Doing better and feeling worse: the political pathology of health policy. In: Knowles JH, ed. Doing better and feeling worse: health in the United States. New York: Norton, 1977:105–123.

8. Stetten DD., Jr. Coping with blindness. N Engl J Med. 1981; 305:458–460.

9. Mechanic D. Factors affecting receptivity to innovations in health care delivery among primary care physicians. In: Politics, medicine, and social science. New York: Wiley-Interscience, 1974:69–87.

10. Goldman L. Factors related to physicians' medical and political attitudes: a documentation of intraprofessional variations. J Health Soc Behav. 1974; 15:177–187.

11. Glaser, WA. Paying the doctor: systems of remuneration and their effects. Baltimore: Johns Hopkins U Press, 1970.

12. Colombotos J, Kirchner C, Millman M. Physicians view national health insurance: a national study. Med Care. 1975; 13:369–396.

8

The Transformation of
Health Providers

AFTER TINKERING AT THE MARGINS of health provision and organization for some years, with only halfhearted efforts to attack core causes and difficulties, the determination of the Congress, state government, and the federal branch reflects a new seriousness. State legislators and federal policymakers are responding, but often with insufficient examination of the unintended effects likely to accompany many of the crude interventions being contemplated. The medical sector is complex and diverse, with strong and sophisticated actors having an important stake in regulatory decisions. These actors now extend beyond the traditional providers and intermediaries to large multihospital chains, suppliers of sophisticated medical technologies, and a growing array of private entrepreneurs. This new constellation contributes increasing uncertainty since the conventional coalitions and rules of the game are less clear, and new interests challenge traditional ones in prestige and power, political access, and sophisticated expertise.

My concern here is with the ethical implications of the transformations taking place. To the patient, the major concerns are access, choice of options, and some assurance of responsive and competent care. Physicians and other health professionals are concerned about protection of their discretion, professional autonomy, and economic security. We should explore Paul Starr's hypothesis[1] that the largest threat to the character of medical practice is neither government involvement nor technical change, but more fundamentally, the emergence of multihospital corporations that have the size, political power, and profit motivation to dictate patterns of practice in a fashion never contemplated by government. We must also consider how the modification of regulatory approaches and reimbursement procedures for professionals, providers, and institutions affects the allocation of health resources, the distribution of benefits among varying population groups, and our concepts of equity.

Implicit in how we structure reimbursement and cost-control efforts are value assumptions about which groups in the population should have priority, which providers should be favored, preferable contexts for the provision of care (whether in doctors' offices, homes, or other community institutions), and the relative importance of prevention, treatment, caring, and curing. The major ethical choices lie less in the definition of death, the dilemma of how aggressively to treat, and patients' rights to have or refuse treatments—the usual subjects of ethical discussion—and more in the mundane financial, organizational, and regulatory incentives and constraints we use.

The most profound choices we face in the decades before us are not the management of new and amazing technologies such as Positron Emission Tomography or diagnostic Nuclear Magnetic Resonance Spectrometry, but rather how we manage sickness, disability, and functioning in old age. The choices we make about the appropriate balance between narrow medical and sociomedical services, promotion of functioning versus traditional care, and institutional and home treatment will affect large numbers of our citizens in extraordinary ways.

But such ethical problems are not resolved in a vacuum. The choices we make have enormous implications for the economic status of professions, the vitality and survival of different types of institutions, and the financial success of major corporations. Having a major stake in how these issues are resolved, such interests occupy a central place in the public discussion of priorities and mechanisms. They do so with political access, technical expertise, and considerable impact on the opinion-making process, and they typically exercise a disproportionate influence on the initiatives we take. This may be inevitable, but it puts a special obligation on the public sector to speak for those population groups most in need, that are dispersed, and that lack the skills, access, and expertise to speak effectively on their own behalf.

The Physician-Patient Relationship

Underlying many of the ethical issues we face in health are inequalities in power and dependence. At the most basic level, differences in knowledge and position of the typical patient and physician, and the exaggerated dependency associated with serious illness, require a great deal of trust. While there is a long history and ethical tradition for negotiating trust between patient and physician, changes in demographics, organization, and technology strain this relationship in fundamental ways. Inequalities in power and dependence and the fragility of trust can also affect many health transactions between physician and nurse, professional and institution, and institution and state authority.

How then are inequalities in knowledge, status, and power effectively managed, and what mechanisms best promote trust? The ability to exercise alternatives—to choose—is basic. Patients feel less vulnerable when they can choose their own provider, site of care, and mode of treatment. Although such choice is often more theoretical than real, it both strengthens the patient's position within the system and deters some abuses. Traditional concepts of doctor-patient relationships view the patient as freely choosing a physician who acts as his or her agent relative to other parties. In theory, patients in the fee-for-service sector, if dissatisfied, can seek care elsewhere. Although location, geographic distribution of facilities and personnel, and other factors, such as the patient's dependency, may inhibit real exercise of choice even when the patient is profoundly dissatisfied, the fact is that many patients can go elsewhere. Similarly, in the case of many HMOs and different types of insurance programs, many consumers have dual choice providing options if they are dissatisfied. Dual choice provisions have a double function, not only allowing a dissatisfied consumer to change plans, but also protecting health programs from dissatisfied clients who may be better served elsewhere.

From Advocating to Allocating

Current efforts to control the escalation of costs often involve modification of two basic conditions of traditional trusting doctor-
patient relationships. First, they often seek to lock in care to a particular category of providers or to restrict choice to a provider who
becomes a gatekeeper to more specialized and expensive services.
Second, they modify the definition of the provider's role as sole agent
of the patient's welfare to a role of balancing the patient's wants and
needs against the aggregate population and a fixed budget. The physician or hospital role, thus, is transformed from *advocating* to *allocating*. Such transformations are inherent in capitation, rate
regulation, and diagnosis-related group methodologies.

The theory of provider-patient relationships does not necessarily
describe the reality. Economic or personal interests of providers and
the limitations of patients' resources did significantly limit treatment
possibilities. But the theory—while only partially true—set a certain
tone. As we look to the future, we should note that existing payment
mechanisms in health care are generally exceptions to those used elsewhere in the economy. Few sectors of our economy draw from an
open-ended fund without budgetary controls, and maximize the
range and quantity of services or products that are provided. Every
other institution is required, whether by the press of competitors or
the limitations of budgets, to make choices, establish priorities, and
use resources in the most effective way. But a constrained budget,
without mechanisms for intelligent choice and without sensitivity to
the complex differentiation among types of health needs and services, opens innumerable perverse possibilities.

The use of DRGs under Medicare suggests some possible dangers. Its application to a single payer, however large the Medicare
program, invites significant cost shifting. By its application to only
a single site of care, it provides opportunities for manipulation in
admission policies, diagnostic practices, patient selection, and pattern of services that will be exceedingly difficult to intelligently monitor, manage, or control. Applied nationwide, DRGs are not as likely
to be fully sensitive to the managerial capacities of hospitals, the true
differentiation in sophistication and quality of services, and the varying missions and practices characteristic of HMOs, teaching hospitals, and other special types of medical care programs. DRGs provide
opportunities to manipulate the payment system without a clear con-

cept of the consequences and how they can be managed intelligently. Unless linked with highly effective utilization and quality assessment, DRGs may reward the shoddy and unscrupulous, while penalizing those who are most honest and effective. They may also alter the shifting patterns of influence between physicians and institutions.

From a federal perspective the motivation in instituting DRGs is clear. Unable or unwilling to politically impose a fully capitated system applying to all basic medical services, DRGs represent the first step in a system that ultimately will expand to other payers and other contexts. It also provides a mechanism to "tighten the screws" should events require such action. As with many policy initiatives in the past several decades, I believe we would have done better to avoid entering this arena through the back door. It would have been more fruitful to correct the system as a whole, and not in a piecemeal fashion.

Cost containment is, of course, a necessity. Many mechanisms, however, can serve the same economic purpose. But alternative mechanisms have varying effects on the internal dynamics of clinics, hospitals, and medical care programs, and provide different incentives for types of care, mix of providers, and the hierarchy of patient care priorities. But even then, the financial structure is only one of several factors that shape the character of care, its distribution in relationship to need, and the balance between discrete technical and other types of services.

Centralized or Individual Authority?

A core question is deciding where the authority to define the appropriate allocation of medical resources available at the national level properly lies. Should the mix of technologies, services, and providers be specified at centralized levels, or are these issues best worked out at the service level in the transactions between patients and doctors, professionals and institutions, and institutions and governmental agencies? Obviously, we will have some mix, but it still remains to be seen in what directions the system tilts.

The issue is difficult in theory and even more so politically, since there are important advantages to each approach. Only centralized authority can make scientifically based allocations using as a basis for such decisions knowledge arising from sophisticated technology assessment, randomized controlled clinical trials, cost-benefit analyses, and sophisticated modeling. Individual professionals, in contrast, are guided much more by their clinical experience and impressions and are extraordinarily immune to any estimates based on aggregate data. The clinical mind-set, whatever it advantages, is often irrational when viewed from a more global perspective. Clinicians tend to believe what they see, but where one sits often distorts one's view. A second advantage of more centralized decision-making is that it avoids forcing the clinician into the role of adjudicating the patient's needs versus those of society.

We cannot assume that professionals, simply left to their own devices, will necessarily be directed by the patient's interests. It is human to have preferences, to pursue the interesting as compared with the dull, and to seek activities and practices held in higher esteem by one's peers and the world at large. It is not clear that physicians, health administrators, and other professionals would allocate resources in direct relationship to need as compared with the attractiveness and sophistication of the patient, the inherent challenge and excitement of varying procedures, career needs, and personal inclination.

But strengthening centralized medical authority also carries extraordinary risks. Illness and behavior are complex and uncertain. The process of care is characterized by innumerable biological contingencies, cultural differences, personal preferences, and social situations. It is difficult to conceive of any medical authority, however sophisticated and humane, that has the capacity to do more than set a general framework for such complex transactions. No social policy can be sufficiently sophisticated to anticipate and make provision for the inevitable cases that depart from the norm. Moreover, centralized authority, however benevolent, is isolated from the pain, worry, uncertainty, and disruption that characterize serious illness. It too easily loses touch with the feelings of participants and the tone of interaction. The result is often perverse.

How then do we protect, enhance, and even promote the ethical basis of medical care as a humane calling responsive to the deepest anxieties, fears, and uncertainties of the population? It is not romantic to maintain the government has responsibility not only to insure access to our least fortunate citizens and to set the overall rules of allocation, but also to promote the deeper meaning of medicine as an institution that preserves personal and social integration, that nurtures the health of the young and promotes the functioning of the old, that sustains people in distress, and that offers hope and solace as well as science to the seriously ill.

These outcomes cannot be mandated by centralized authority. They can only be facilitated by an equitable framework of allocation that promotes the opportunities for conscientious professionals to do their best within the limits of their knowledge and resources. This can only be accomplished by building a framework of trust at the level of doctor-patient contact and a framework of equity at the societal level. The government's proper concern for cost and determinations of what proportion of public budgets should be allocated to health can be accomplished by a capitation approach, and public policy needs can be met without clinical intrusions. Capitation is a highly flexible payment mechanism that can be weighted by physician characteristics, patient characteristics, and unique features of specific geographic areas. Internationally, there is vast experience and knowledge on the conceptual, administrative, and regulatory aspects of this approach.

Responsibility of the Medical Profession

If government is not to intrude in clinical affairs while paying the bill, much responsibility rests on the profession of medicine and other professional groups. If the system is to work, these professionals must assume group, as well as individual, responsibility and adopt both informal and formal means to protect against fraud, deception, and wastefulness. Three objectives must be satisfied. First, variations in medical practice that cannot be justified by clinical uncertainty or differences in patient populations must be intelligently constrained. This requires effective and informed peer review. While we cannot feel confident that professionals will seriously police one another in a broad sense, there is more likelihood that this can take place in the carefully defined domain of resource allocation and use. To the extent that professionals understand that they must exercise group responsibility that goes beyond concern about their own patients, significant accomplishments are possible.

A second objective it to develop incentives for the types of care we believe should be emphasized. Physicians in each specialty, for example, earn a great deal more for each hour they spend in hospital work as compared with ambulatory care. Average office-based physicians can earn 50 to 60 per cent more per hour spent in hospital care than in their offices, and the types of inputs used in hospitals per hour of physician time may cost twice as much as those used in office-based practice. Is this the pattern of care we wish to encourage? Means must also be developed to insure that resources are allocated fairly and not disproportionately to the most attractive, aggressive, sophisticated, or demanding patient.

The third objective is the most difficult one to achieve because it involves the complexities of interpersonal relations and differences in culture, values, and modes of personal negotiation. When physicians work within fixed budgets and are paid indirectly by salary or capitation and not directly by the patient, even greater effort than usual is required to encourage sensitive and equitable care. Physicians as peers, rather than external authority, are the most legitimate sources of such encouragement. Physicians as a group must develop nonmonetary reward systems that substitute for the big fee.

Efforts to develop a broader range of incentives, coupled with consumer choice and meaningful opportunities for grievance resolution without resort to litigation, offer at least a meaningful framework for addressing ethical requirements of the new era. The history of the profession in these areas is less than encouraging, and many are skeptical that much can be accomplished without forceful outside regulatory authority. Believing that the heavy hand of government causes more problems than it solves, I hope very much that the professions can constructively address these issues. My message should be clear. Administrative rationing of medical care is neither desirable nor inevitable. It will come, however, unless health professionals see the urgency of their responsibility, not only for moderating their own behaviors, but also for the functioning of the health sector as a whole. There are complications, of course. The growing number of doctors, antitrust regulations, and the complexity of legislation and litigation affecting practice all highlight the care with which these tasks must be undertaken. We will all benefit to the extent that the professions work constructively to develop internal mechanisms consistent with social need and good patient care. The next chapter provides one such example.

References

1. Starr P. The social transformation of American medicine. New York: Basic Books, 1982:514.

9

A Cooperative Agenda
for Medicine and Nursing

THE INTERFACE between medicine and nursing has become a frequent topic of debate and has captured broad public interest.[1] The recent debate has focused on nurses' increasing dissatisfaction with hospital practice, including their relationships with physicians. Physicians have raised questions about the appropriate roles for nurses, given the rapid increase in the number of practicing physicians. Unfortunately, the debate has often focused on the diverging interests and competitive strain between nursing and medicine which is unnecessarily exaggerated and diverts attention from the core of health care in which doctors and nurses who work together can promote their mutual interests and those of their patients.

Perspectives of Physicians, Nurses, and Patients

The work of the physician has grown enormously in scope not only because of biomedical advances but also because of the "medicali-

This chapter was coauthored with Linda Aiken.

zation" of everyday problems.[2] Physicians must be aware, as never before, of the technical requirements of their work, but they must also be knowledgeable about diverse psychosocial and behavioral issues. Many physicians deeply resent the growth of regulation and increasing criticism from patients and the mass media. Some fear an erosion of their economic status and clinical autonomy.[3] Most are searching for ways of being responsive while maintaining their own views of how medicine should be practiced.

A key issue is how physicians, faced with multiple and sometimes conflicting expectations, can cope constructively with the stresses of their role and also meet the requirement that they remain technically expert while maintaining a humane attitude toward patients and a broad view of their problems and needs. Successfully achieving this will depend in large part on the arrangments that physicians work out with the members of the other health professions, particularly nursing.

Nursing must be seen within the context of broad social changes in sex roles and in women's conceptions of themselves. The proportion of women in the work force has increased dramatically, and women expect the same opportunities, incentives, and rewards that men receive for performing comparable jobs.[4] An increasing number of women plan to spend their adult lives in the work force and are seeking opportunities for growth and development through their employment. They are increasingly dissatisfied with episodic work, with an absence of rewards and career ladders, and with expectations that they will be deferential and perform tasks not relevant to work that are not expected of men. With heightened aspirations, women are now entering the professions in greatly increased numbers. Women who in earlier times might have chosen nursing, social work, or teaching are now becoming physicians, lawyers, and business executives.

Nursing exemplifies many of the limitations of "women's occupations" and women's changing career expectations. The growing knowledge base and technical demands of nursing care and the plain hard work in terms of physical labor, night and weekend work hours, social stress, and continuing responsibility are poorly remunerated in comparison to other occupations demanding similar levels of education, skill, and responsibility. The income gap between nurses and physicians, for example, has increased dramatically since 1945. After World War II, nurses' incomes were one-third of physicians' incomes, but by 1980 nurses were earning less than one-fifth as much as doctors.[5] Moreover, the existing salary structures do not reward experienced, career-oriented nurses.Beginning nurses who are just out of school earn only slightly less than nurses with years of clinical experience.[6] The loss of experienced nurses, partly a result of inadequate remuneration, leaves younger nurses without the support necessary to cope with responsibilities that can easily overwhelm them.

Given the poor economic rewards for becoming and remaining a nurse, nonmonetary rewards are very important in maintaining nurses' career commitments and morale. Nurses have lacked the authority to make many simple decisions necessary for the safety and comfort of patients, and they have been expected to defer to medical authority,[7] even in situations in which they possess greater experience. The undervaluation of their knowledge and experience is a major source of nurses' dissatisfaction and frustration with their current roles.

Patients generally believe that their physicians are technically competent. Satisfaction depends on access to services and on the degree to which physicians avoid a sense of haste, allow patients to ask questions, and provide responsive and informative feedback. Most dissatisfaction is evident among chronically ill patients and their families who face long periods of uncertainty and debility. The frustration that they experience often reflects the difficulties of gaining sufficient information and advice. Physicians, in coordinating hospital work with office-based practice, often cannot arrange their schedules to coincide with the times when families are usually present in the hospital. These problems can be minimized and frequently avoided through more effective collaboration between doctors and nurses. In considering means of effective collaboration, we will discuss the care of patients in hospitals and nursing homes.

Patient Care in Hospitals and Nursing Homes

Over the past 10 years technologic advances and changes in patterns of medical practice have markedly altered the nature of hospital care. The average length of a hospital stay has been reduced by 20 per cent since 1970. More services can be given in a shorter period, and the diagnostic case-mix has shifted toward a sicker group of patients.[8] The number of intensive care beds increased by more than 74 per cent between 1972 and 1980.[9,10]

More complex technology, a greater need for services among hospitalized patients, and more difficult problems of coordinating the growing number of specialized personnnel involved in caring for patients put major responsibilities and stresses on nurses. These demands are exacerbated when physicians who have formal authority are absent from patient care settings because of other responsibilities and changing work habits.

The number of hours worked by the average physician has declined from over 65 hours a week in 1943[11] to less than 50 hours a week in 1980.[12] Moreover, most physicians spend less than two hours a day in making rounds in the hospital.[13] Thus, while patients are more acutely ill than ever before, there are extended periods during which physicians are not present in the hospital or easily accessible for direct consultation. Nurses are left with the continuing responsibility for acutely ill patients, but their authority to act in the absence of the physician has not been formally modified.

The realities of hospital practice have meant that nurses have become more directly involved in patient treatment. In fact, many of the tasks formerly regarded as solely those of physicians are now commonly shared by nurses. Monitoring cardiac arrhythmias, electrolytes, and blood gases and administration of intravenous medication are but a few of many examples. This shifting interface between nurses and physicians has caused some confusion about the proper role for nurses and the relation of nursing functions to medical functions in the optimal care of patients. In intensive care units and various specialty services in which the interface has been well-defined and timely decision-making is critical, physicians and nurses have worked together effectively and without conflict. The dramatically increased survival rates of low-birth-weight infants, for example, are directly attributable both to advanced knowledge and technology and to the effective collaboration of doctors and nurses.

However, in noncritical care, the authority of nurses to make necessary decisions is more ambiguous. This is not a problem of confrontation involving boundary disputes; nurses do not seek to be the "captain of the team." They do, however, need the authority to act in matters within their spheres of competence. Changing inappropriate special diets; modifying medications when indicated, including dosage and mode of administration; rescheduling strenuous diagnostic procedures as warranted by patients' conditions; changing surgical dressings if needed; deciding on the frequency of vital-sign monitoring; inserting catheters for patients unable to void; and contributing to decisions on the appropriate time and place for hospital discharge are all examples of such judgments, which if not made in a timely fashion result in inconvenience and discomfort to patients and in diminished productivity for both doctors and nurses.

Hospitalized patients have a variety of needs related to their illnesses and to their overall well-being that may be as important to the ultimate outcome as specific medical interventions. Important from a social perspective is determining the least restrictive treatment regimen and teaching patients to manage their lives to minimize illness-related disabilities and to cope with various contingencies and uncertainties. Patients need opportunities to ask questions, to experiment with aspects of the treatment regimen, and to obtain informative and supportive feedback. When a variety of medical and other health personnel are involved in the patient's hospital care, there is a further need for effective and consistent communication with the patient and with staff to minimize contradictions, duplication of efforts, unnecessary anxieties, and confusions and breakdowns in the process of care. Nurses can be extraordinarily helpful in these areas.

Nursing homes are a major source of national concern.[14] Unfortunately, neither medicine nor nursing has assumed a leadership role in improving these institutions, which care for a larger number of patients each day than our entire community hospital system. Only 17 per cent of physicians participate in nursing home care at all.[15] Primary care physicians, who are expected to shoulder most of the burden of nursing home coverage, spend on the average less than $1\frac{1}{2}$ hours a month caring for their patients in nursing homes, whereas subspecialists spend less than 30 minutes a month.[13] In reality, physicians alone are not likely to make a real difference in nursing homes; they simply are not present for long enough periods.

In contrast, nurses are in nursing homes every day, and most of what is required there is nursing, not medical care. This continuity of contact allows nurses to assess each patient's potential and to plan care that enhances individual strengths. Many of the procedures that are often performed in nursing homes and that foster dependency, including overmedication, restraints, and unnecessary use of Foley catheters for incontinence, can be avoided by well-planned and supervised care. In addition, nurses with the appropriate clinical skills and with consultative relationships with physicians could considerably reduce the unnecessary use of costly emergency-room and hospital inpatient services by nursing home patients, by giving greater attention to prevention and providing more timely identification of acute problems that are likely to become more severe over time.

A promising strategy for the improvement of nursing home care is to strengthen the role of nurses as primary providers, and physicians in consultative roles. Physicians and nurses working collaboratively could improve care for patients, enhance opportunities for recruitment and retention of nurses, and give physicians a greater sense of accomplishment about the value of their own participation in nursing home care.

Opportunities or Constraints: A Cooperative Agenda

The current attention paid to physician-nurse relationships is in part influenced by the growing physician supply and by perceptions of economic competition. Such fears are exaggerated by the focus on nurse practitioners. The acute threat posed by 20,000 nurse practitioners within a pool of more than 1 million practicing nurses, and compared with 450,000 doctors, is more symbolic than real. For nurses, the dominant workplace is the hospital or nursing home, and in these contexts physicians and nurses are neither in serious boundary disputes nor in competition for the same dollars. Since nurses' remuneration derives from the hospital or nursing home charge per diem, whereas physicians' incomes are primarily fee-for-service, gains for nurses are unlikely to affect the economic status of physicians.

Nurses primarily support and complement medical care. The expanded clinical responsibilities of nurses have freed physicians to perform medical functions that require their unique expertise and that tend to more remunerative than most functions that nurses perform. Nurses also provide important added dimensions of care that are too often neglected in busy institutional settings. However, their authority to make clinical decisions needs to be redefined in the light of their changing responsibilities and increased competence. To do this, serious attention must be given to developing a differentiated nursing structure that clearly identifies nurses according to their levels of expertise. Physicians often do not feel confident in delegating complex tasks that require difficult judgments to nurses, among whom they cannot clearly differentiate the more educated or experienced. Nurse staffing patterns in hospitals must also be reorganized to allow nurses ongoing responsibility for defined groups of patients. The value of nursing services to patients and to physicians is severely compromised when continuity of contact with patients is discouraged by moving nurses from one service to another.

Nurses are very versatile. They can move competently among many roles in hospital settings, from intensive care to ward management. However, this apparent advantage is one of nursing's key weaknesses, contributing to a host of problems, including lack of continuity of care. The unique contributions and experiences of nurses are sometimes undervalued, and they are required to perform a wide variety of functions that could be done by others. Such use decreases productivity, creates apparent shortages, and may even debase the professional skills and value of more experienced nurses.[5]

Hospitals increasingly face caps and restrictive budgets, and these types of constraints are likely to become more common. Cost-containment policies clearly increase competitive tensions among the health professions and constrain the wages of nurses paid through the hospital's or nursing home's per diem charges. But cost-containment concerns also focus attention on how quality of care can be maintained while expenditures are limited.

Nurses can assist physician groups in conserving time and resources and allow a more efficient response to patient's needs. However, physicians must also be sensitive to the economic requirements necessary to maintain the skilled nursing staff on which they depend so heavily. Physicians and hospital managers will undoubtedly be faced in the future with setting priorities regarding the allocation of resources within hospitals, and one of the trade-offs is likely to be equipment and capital expenditures versus investment in professional personnel—including nurses.

Among the issues requiring examination is how hospitals can limit turnover among nurses to avoid wasteful expenditures. The estimated average annual turnover rate of hospital nurses nationwide is 30 per cent. Hospitals spent an average of $768 in 1981 to hire each new nurse,[16] and many hospitals also sponsor expensive supervised in-service training programs for each entry-level nurse employed.[17]

Thus, nurse turnover may be adding as much as several million dollars a year to national health expenditures. If hospitals could attract and retain experienced nurses who would assume greater responsibility for coordination of efforts and resources, many inefficient and redundant efforts could be avoided. The trade-offs between the necessary added expenditures for career grades in nursing and the resultant savings need to be evaluated. A substantial body of evidence now indicates that fewer experienced nurses can manage a unit more efficiently than many more transitory personnel or those with fewer skills who require continued supervision.[18]

High-quality nursing care depends on the talent pool from which nurses are drawn and retention of the most skilled and experienced nurses in clinical settings. Nursing increasingly competes with a wide range of career choices for talented recruits. The development of a stable and rewarding career structure is important both for revitalizing the entry pool and maintaining nurses' career commitments, and is an issue that should be high on the agenda for both medicine and nursing.

Probably the most important factor contributing to poor physician-nurse relationships is a lack of understanding between both groups about the kinds of problems each faces. Ironically, as the complexities of medical care have increased, making the collaboration of doctors and nurses more critical in achieving good patient outcomes, medical schools and nursing schools have become increasingly isolated from one another. Nursing students need closer involvement with the changing medical science base and with new medical technologies. Medical students could profit from the strong social and behavioral orientations in nursing and the emphasis on improving patients' levels of function—physical and social. Clearly, medical schools and nursing schools should be more closely linked academically, and this should be a major item on their joint agenda.

In addition, education for future patterns of practice requires a reinforcing context. A key factor is the presence of senior physicians and nurses who demonstrate by their own behavior their commitment to a stronger partnership. Models are needed to build from the early interaction in which the young house officer is assisted by the experienced nurse in "learning the ropes." A promising strategy for increasing partnership models is for university nurse faculty to practice in teaching hospitals. A professor of nursing who would be the counterpart of the physician chief of each clinical service is needed.

Collaboration between medical and nursing faculty in practice, clinical research, and teaching could be a potent force in improving both patient care and the education of young doctors and nurses.

To summarize, although the interests of medicine and nursing diverge in some areas, there is a considerable mutual interest in the central aspects of patient care. Reimbursement of nurses is not in direct competition with physicians' incomes, and the interests of medicine and patient care would be served by a differentiated nursing career structure that properly recognized the value of accumulated skill and experience. Medical schools and nursing schools should develop closer academic ties to improve the education of both doctors and nurses and to set the stage for more effective collaboration in the future.

References

1. National Commission on Nursing. Summary of the public hearings. Chicago: American Hospital Association, 1981.
2. Fox RC. The medicalization and demedicalization of American society. In: Knowles JR, ed. Doing better and feeling worse: health in the United States. New York: Norton, 1977:9–22.
3. Louis Harris and Associates. Medical practice in the 1980s: physicians look at their changing profession. Study no. 804015. New York: Louis Harris and Associates, 1981.
4. Treiman DJ, Hartmann HI, eds. Women, work, and wages: equal pay for jobs of equal value. Washington, D.C.: National Academy Press, 1981.
5. Aiken LH, Blendon RJ, Rogers DE. The shortage of hospital nurses: a new perspective. Ann Intern Med. 1981; 95:365–72.
6. Donovan L. Survey of nursing incomes. Part 2. What increases income most? RN. 1980; 43:27–30.
7. Stein LI. The doctor-nurse game. Arch Gen Psychiatry. 1967; 16:699–703.
8. National Center for Health Statistics. Health United States, 1980: Hyattsville, Md: Natonal Center for Health Statistics, 1980. (DHEW publication no. [PHS] 81–1232).
9. American Hospital Association. Hospital statistics, 1972. Chicago: American Hospital Association, 1972:205, 208.
10. *Idem.* Hospital statistics, 1981. Chicago: American Hospital Association, 1981:206–207.

11. Physicians economic status. Med Econ. 1944; 22(2):49.
12. Glandon GL, Werner JL. Physician's practice experience during the decade of the 1970s. JAMA. 1980; 244:2514–2518.
13. The Robert Wood Johnson Foundation. Medical practice in the United States: a special report. Princeton, NJ.: The Robert Wood Johnson Foundation, 1982:34–35.
14. Vladeck BC. Unloving care: the nursing home tragedy. New York: Basic Books, 1980.
15. Smits HL. Manpower for long-term care: two simple suggestions. Nat J. 1981; 13:807–809.
16. National Association of Nurse Recruiters, Recruitment survey. Pitman, N.J.: National Association of Nurse Recruiters, 1981.
17. White CH. Redefining professional nursing: solution to the chronic shortage? Hosp Prog. 1981; 62(10):40–46.
18. Aiken LH, ed. Nursing in the 1980s: crises, opportunities, challenges. Philadelphia: Lippincott, 1982.

PART IV

The Health of Special Populations

10

Social Factors Affecting the Mental Health of the Elderly

THROUGHOUT THE DEVELOPED WORLD, elderly persons are a growing proportion of the population, and in many countries the number of very old persons is increasing markedly. In the United States, for example, the number of elderly increased 55 per cent between 1960 and 1980 to almost 30 million. By the year 2000, we expect an elderly population of more than 36 million. More dramatic and important for health policy, however, is that between 1960 and 1980, persons over 85 years of age increased 174 per cent, and this population is expected to increase an additional 110 per cent between 1980 and the end of the century.[1] By the year 2000, one-quarter of the elderly population will be older than 80. These trends toward an aging population are even more pronounced in various European nations.[2] Social expenditures as a proportion of gross national product has grown remarkably in all European nations between 1960 and 1981, and has brought about reassessments and retrenchment affecting the elderly.[3]

The age structure of the population is a product of the fertility of various population cohorts in the past and improving longevity throughout the life course. The increasing numbers and proportions of the elderly of various ages reflect the fact that fertility has remarkably decreased in developed nations with more education, changing family norms, and contraceptive technologies; while improved social conditions, life-styles, and medical interventions have extended the expected life span and period of effective functioning.

The age structure of populations, and the number of people in successive cohorts, have important impact on the opportunities and frustrations experienced by the individuals who make up these cohorts. As the proportion of retired elderly increases in a population relative to those working, a smaller proportion of the population must support the social security, medical care, and welfare benefits of the retired or nonworking population. As these demands fall on smaller segments of populations, potentialities arise for inadequate provision for the elderly and increased conflict among generations. Such problems are not inevitable. They depend on the strength of the economy, the values of the society, and the political power of the elderly, among other factors.[4]

In examining the health and welfare of the elderly, and their psychological vulnerability, one must differentiate between age and historical cohort.[5] Each age cohort faces unique social, economic, and health issues over the life span that shapes personal development, coping resources, and physical functioning. In relation to health, for example, it is abundantly clear that a person of age 65, 75, or even 80 is much more likely than in the past to remain healthy, to live an active and satisfying life, and to retain skills and social effectiveness.[6] The artificial dichotomy of those above and below age 65, although socially important because of retirement policies, pension rights, and social security benefits, have little scientific relevance for understanding vulnerability and risk. Moreover, health outcomes of past cohorts, when used to project the future burden of illness, health care needs, and dependency, while informative, must be used with sensitivity and care.

While aging is not the same as morbidity or loss of capacities, it is significantly correlated with such risks. While we remain uncertain as to whether increasing length of life will be relatively free of serious disease until the approach of death,[7] or marked by high rates of illness burden, incapacity, and dependence over some considerable time,[8] the fact is that with increased scientific knowledge, improved technology, high expectations among the elderly, and their growing political influence, demands for health and social security programs will become a difficult challenge for most developed societies.

While we often think of the aged as a frail subgroup, the majority of aged persons are resilient.[9] This reflects partly selective mortality and partly the fact that many of the same social, environmental, and personal factors that promote effective functioning in young adulthood and middle age continue throughout the life span. High-quality epidemiological data are limited, and major problems involving measurement and nosology persist, but most studies suggest that the incidence of psychiatric impairments, in contrast to chronic physical illness, is modest in the elderly relative to other age groups.[10-12] The prevalence, of course, may be higher because of the longevity of patients with intractable mental disorders that occur at younger ages but persist or recur in later life. Organic brain syndromes, and particularly senile dementia of the Alzheimer's type (SDAT), pose major challenges in old age[13] both in appropriate diagnosis and the provision of humane care.

The factors promoting vulnerability and risk of psychiatric disorder among the elderly are similar to those among younger populations, but various risk factors, or those affecting the course of disease, may be more exaggerated among the elderly. One of the most consistent factors associated with psychiatric morbidity, for example, is deprived socioeconomic status, and in most nations the elderly are at greater risk of deprivation of income and a valued social position. Given the large differential in mortality by sex, large numbers of widows in single-person dwellings must struggle to make ends meet. Socioeconomic deficiencies may affect the quality of shelter, nutrition, social participation, household assistance, and acquistion of needed medical care. Although the economic position of the elderly has been enhanced enormously by improvements in social security, and various health and social programs, many elderly still experience considerable deprivations that interact with other social and biological factors contributing to distress and disorder. One irony is that as income improves, elderly persons choose to live alone, and this decision makes it less likely that they will have an adequate living standard or the assistance that helps functioning in the community.[2]

Most studies show that elderly persons continue active relationships with children and kin, but these increasingly are independent of multigeneration households. While elderly persons living by themselves receive assistance and nurturance from loved ones, such assistance is relatively uncertain as friends, relatives, and even children themselves confront life problems, age, and die. What may have once been an effective and strong source of help and social support may erode with the aging process, and the elderly if they are to retain their independence and avoid institutionalization may require formal community and home care services that are too often fragmentary, underdeveloped, and unresponsive.

Residence of the elderly depends on their income, cultural attitudes toward household composition, housing availability, number and geographic mobility of children, and beliefs about financial responsibility of children who themselves may be retired or approaching retirement. In developed countries, children of the elderly, and the aged themselves, see the primary responsibility for the economic welfare of the aged as resting with government and the social security system. Between 1957 and 1974, the proportion of the public considering children responsible for income support of the elderly in the United States decreased from 53 to 10 percent, and the elderly themselves have even lower expectations.[2] Similar patterns are found in other Western countries, as in Holland, where one survey found that less than 10 per cent of old people considered children responsible for financial support of the elderly. In some developed countries, Japan for example, elderly are much more likely to live with their children, but even this pattern appears to be weakening with relief of housing shortages and changes in attitudes and work force participation.

Good physical health, of course, is a major asset, and when combined with adequate economic resources and social support, provide the basis for a continuing life of satisfaction and well-being among the elderly. Chronic physical illness that induces disability and restricts desired activity, in contrast, is a source of dissatisfaction, depression, and diminished well-being. Moreover, medication for chronic conditions, and their multiple interactive effects, may further diminish a sense of vitality. Recent studies suggest hypersensitivity of the elderly to many drugs and that the elderly suffer from both overmedication and poor compliance. They also indicate that in the United States almost three-quarters of the elderly population received a prescription outside the hospital in 1977, and those who received at least one prescription averaged 14.2 during the year.[14]

While certain physical and perceptual capacities diminish with aging, many studies suggest that the stereotype of a downward course in cognitive and social performance is simplistic and ignores both the heterogeneity of the aged and the range of judgmental and coping skills that develop over the life course.[15,16] Many elderly persons continue to develop their social and coping capacities and others suffer decrements due as much to social and community attitudes as incapacities to perform. Older persons tend to be less physically strong, slower in response, and more cautious and concerned about responding correctly but may counterbalance these with more mature judgment and broader experience. The social response, however, is frequently impatient and may reinforce and stigmatize small deficits that undermine self-esteem, confidence, and a desire for continued participation. These in turn may adversely affect satisfaction and well-being.

The importance of activity and continued participation for maintaining individual skills and overall competence cannot be overemphasized. One of the important conclusions derived from many studies of mental patients is that inactivity and withdrawal promotes secondary disabilities that may be more profound than the initial problem.[17] Inactivity is a significant risk factor for the deterioration of the elderly, and one of the significant preventive insights that can be derived from the literature is the importance of encouraging continued functioning. Experiments involving the elderly that allow their own choices, decision-making, and responsibility are associated with enhanced well-being. In contrast, institutional settings, and even community attitudes and responses, commonly encourage dependence and helplessness among many elderly persons. It would be sad to forget a lesson learned so painfully over many decades in the care of the chronic mental patient and persons with significant physical impairments and illnesses. It is through continued activity that individuals maintain their skills and sense of social value.[18]

There is much evidence, as well, that involvement in and commitment to a community or system of cherished values promotes health and well-being.[19] Individuals more closely integrated into family, neighborhood, and community, and who are less alienated and anomic, live longer and express greater well-being. There are many ways in which modern societies make the elderly feel redundant and prematurely limit their options for meaningful activities. Correction of discrimination and stigmatization of the aged can do a great deal to enhance well-being.

Coping effectiveness and self-confidence, in part, depend on confronting familiar challenges that have been mastered successfully in the past. Various epidemiological studies suggest that rapid social change and social instability pose readjustment problems that all individuals, and perhaps the elderly most of all, find difficult. In the current conceptualization, instability is measured by adverse life events, and there is mounting evidence that such events, in the absence of strong coping skills and social supports, may overwhelm the individual resulting in distress and behavioral dysfunction, physical illness, or both.[20] Among the elderly, such results are seen particularly in males following the death of their spouses, although widows appear to cope more effectively and do not show comparable adverse effects. Disorientation and increased mortality also appears to be associated with moving elderly persons from familiar to unfamiliar environments, such as from home to institution or from one institution to another. While we have yet to identify the specific intervening variables that increase risk, studies of many populations, using diverse methods and approaches, support the general hypothesis that rapid change, even if it brings positive and valued benefits, may have negative consequences for physical functioning and health.

The types of broad influences I have described—such as material welfare, the maintenance and enhancement of coping skills, the nurturance of intimacy and social ties, involvement in and commitment to a system of cherished values, and social stability—may affect health directly but also influence such essential psychological dispositions as hope and optimism, self-esteem and confidence, and motivation for maintaining participation in activities. These attitudinal and behavioral dispositions, in turn, affect perceptions of physical health and well-being; complaints of depression, anxiety, and somatic discomforts; and use of medical, psychological, and social services.[21] They also increase vulnerability to illness and disability; delay recovery from serious physical illness, surgery, and hospitalization; and may also adversely influence essential health behavior and self-care, including nutrition, use of alcohol and palliative drugs, and exercise and physical activity important for health maintenance.

Social Factors Affecting the Care of the Elderly

The ability of the elderly to live in the community, to receive appropriate medical and social care, and to avoid institutionalization depends on social security and health entitlements, the organization of families and households, cultural values, and the preferences of the aged themselves. In the last several decades there has been substantial improvement in social security and welfare systems that have allowed people to leave the work force earlier in their lives and, with increased longevity, has led to a much longer span of retirement prior to death.[22] The growth of state sponsored medical insurance for the elderly has substantially increased their share of the funds invested in medical care and access to medical services.

In the United States, public funding for medical care for the elderly and the poor, and the incentives implicit in the Medicare and Medicaid programs, greatly influenced patterns of care for the elderly and forces toward institutionalization. The availability of new funding through these programs, introduced in the mid-1960s, encouraged a substantial growth of nursing home beds and a narrow medical and institutional orientation to the health problems of the aged. Elderly with long-standing psychiatric problems, and those developing new problems of disorientation and incapacity, were particularly affected since existing programs were overwhelmingly directed to care for services provided in institutions, but severely restricted payments for out-of-hospital mental health services.[23] Because of the financial incentives implicit in these programs, the nursing home became a convenient solution not only for the disoriented or incapacitated elderly, but also for many younger chronic mental patients who had limited alternatives for appropriate care.

In the period 1975–1977, of the 1.3 million nursing home beds, approximately 750,000 were occupied by persons with mental impairments.[24] Approximately 350,000 were persons with a primary or secondary mental health diagnosis based on the International Classification of Disease (ICD), and 400,000 diagnosed as suffering from senility without psychosis. In contrast to the 125,000 chronic patients in mental health institutions, the nursing home was the hidden but primary system of chronic mental health care for patients of all ages. While there were strong doubts that the restrictive and inactive atmospheres of these institutions, their low levels of professional staffing, and their dependence on sedation to manage patients, was a good strategy for care of chronicity,[25] this pattern emerged because existing programs paid for such care and not for alternatives. While most analysts concede that such care is neither cost-effective in the individual case, nor the best available system for caring for many of the patients involved, the advantage of the system relative to alternatives is that it has implicit built-in financial protections. The typical elderly person does much to resist institutionalization, and the nursing home becomes the last resort when other informal mechanisms to retain independence fail. The fear among financial analysts is that a more cost-effective but attractive home care alternative would enlist many more elderly leading to substantially increased aggregate costs.

As we look to the future, it is clear that we need a better way of developing community care structures for the elderly and the chronically mentally ill. Such alternatives are particularly difficult to develop and administrate and to finance under existing health and welfare programs. But they offer better opportunities to promote continued functioning and to avoid dependence, and to provide a wide range of sociomedical services better fitted to the needs of the elderly. The medicalization of long-term care encourages unrealistic curative efforts, overuse of technologies that often contribute to the further incapacity of many frail elderly, and inappropriate heroic efforts.[26] While the appropriate margins of medical activity are not well defined, and good medical care has an indispensable role in the overall pattern, the medical dominance of long-term care and a narrow medical approach can be a real disservice to meeting the health needs of the elderly.

As we confront new demographic realities in the coming decades, there is much we can do to enhance the quality of life of the elderly and to facilitate their continued involvement and contributions to the community. The development of a sound system of social security has been the single most significant factor affecting the welfare of the aged in the United States during this century. While the system faces financial problems at various points in time because of changing demography and economic circumstances, rates of taxation for social welfare benefits are comparatively low in the United States relative to many European nations. Government spending relative to the gross national product was only 33.2 per cent in 1980, as compared with 40.7 per cent in Canada, 46.2 per cent in France, 46.9 per cent in Germany, and 66.7 per cent in Sweden.[27] There is little doubt that the United States can finance an adequate social security system. The seeming alarm is as much a crisis of values as an issue of economic viability.

The foregoing is not to suggest that the changing demographic structures of developed nations do not pose serious problems of equity among varying age cohorts with changes in the dependency ratio between the working population and the elderly. In the United States, for example, there were approximately nine workers for each elderly person in 1930, approximately four expected between 1980 and 2010,[9] and approximately two in 2030 if present trends continue. A substantial improvement in the economic status of the elderly has occurred during this period, closing the gap in economic deprivations between the elderly and other age groups. When one considers need and other nonincome transfers to the aged, they may even be better off economically than some other age groups. But the elderly population is not homogeneous and includes subpopulations that suffer considerable privations.

While the dependency ratio relative to the elderly has been increasing, declining fertility has reduced the total dependency ratio relative to what it was in 1970,[28] and in the aggregate it is expected to decline during the next century. While the economic resources necessary to support an elderly person relative to a child are more substantial, it is increasingly asked whether more of the economic care for the aged should be assumed by their children. Both the fact that the aged's children are themselves increasingly elderly and that the public perceives the aged as a national responsibility, make it questionable that a significant solution can be found in transferring significant costs to their children.

Given the concerns about the growing proportions of elderly relative to the working population, it is ironic that we provide few incentives for the young elderly who retain their motivation and vitality to remain in the work force. Both our social security and tax systems do little to encourage continued participation in work and relatively few efforts are made to utilize the skills, experience, and wisdom of the elderly in voluntary activities. The elderly population constitutes a large untapped reservoir of skill and potential productivity that we have not been particularly imaginative about. Current knowledge suggests that using this resource would also contribute in many ways to the health and vitality of the elderly as well.

In much of the world, we can do a great deal to capitalize on the desire of the elderly themselves to retain function and avoid dependence and particularly institutionalization. Elderly persons commonly tolerate many privations and difficulties to retain residence in their own households and to avoid institutional dependency. Entry into a nursing home or comparable facility often follows major illness and disability, death or major illness of a spouse or primary caretaker, or other major breakdowns in social supports. Institutionalization is resisted and typically is a last resort when individuals can no longer manage by themselves.

The foregoing suggests that sound social policy regarding the aged would make accessible the types of home care and supports that assist the elderly person's struggle to maintain independence and control over their lives. Innumerable studies show that home care is preferred by the elderly and cost-effective on an individual basis. In the aggregate, home care has threatening financial implications because the negative perceptions of nursing homes result in many needy elderly struggling along without services, and the unattractiveness of this alternative effectively operates to ration services and expenditures. The fear is, and it is supported by some evidence, that should more attractive options be available, the demand will rise substantially. Such financial concerns are not trivial, but it would be more appropriate and humane to develop better quality assessment and screening devices for access to long-term care services than to pursue solutions whose primary advantage is that the adversiveness of the service deters demand.

A second important area for action as well as research is the design of incentives that encourage isolated elderly to live together, substantially increasing their financial resources and social supports. While present trends are toward increased single-person households,[2] and many elderly prefer this, creative joint housing arrangements that allow communal living but preserve privacy as well might influence individual decision-making. Moreover, much more could be done to help the elderly identify compatible living partners, and to socially legitimize such household arrangements. We also need to develop more effective structures that capture the energies of the more vigorous elderly to contribute to those more frail or to the society more generally.

Developed societies that anticipate an increasing elderly population have grave concerns about the growing possibilities and costs of medical care, the increasing burden of financing long-term care, and the decreasing proportion of persons in the labor force in relation to the elderly. We must evolve a better method of balancing the allocation of available resources between hospital-based medical care, home-based sociomedical care, and appropriate long-term care where the medical model is not so dominant. One way of achieving this is by developing organizations in the community that assume responsibility for the entire spectrum of services on a capitated basis, that either maintain or contract for all necessary services on behalf of the elderly, and that make determinations of appropriate patterns of care given various needs, inclinations and tastes of those for whom they are responsible. Such community structures face formidable political and technical barriers and much effort would be necessary to develop appropriate criteria and quality assurance measures and to build the organizational structures necessary to bridge the array of professional and supportive services required.

The challenges ahead in the care of the aged are not easy. They make clear the limitations of our resources, the inadequacies of our knowledge, and the fragmentation of our social policies and politics. How we respond to the challenge to provide humane and responsive care to our elderly, and the quality of life and function we allow them in their remaining years, will say much about Western societies and the integrity of their systems of values and behavior.

References

1. Rice D, Feldman J. Living longer in the United States: demographic changes and health needs of the elderly. Health Soc. 1983; 61:362–396.
2. Crystal S. America's old age crisis: public policy and the two worlds of aging. New York: Basic Books, 1982.
3. Markham J. Europe, too, feels the social program pinch. New York Times, February 19, 1984, Sec. E:3.
4. Estes C. Fiscal austerity and aging. In: Estes C, Newcomer R and Associates. Fiscal austerity and aging: shifting government responsibility for the elderly. Beverly Hills, Calif.: Sage, 1983:25.
5. Riley M, Abeles R, Teitelbaum M, eds. Aging from birth to death: vol II, sociotemporal perspectives. Boulder, Colo.: Westview Press, 1982:1–26.
6. Feldman J. Work ability of the aged under conditions of improving mortality. Health Soc. 1983; 61:430–444.
7. Fries JF. Aging, natural death, and the compression of morbidity. N Engl J Med. 1980; 303:130–135.
8. Schneider E, Brody J. Aging, natural death, and the compression of morbidity: another view. N Engl J Med. 1983; 309:854–855.
9. National Research on Aging Planning Panel. Toward an independent old age: a national plan for research on aging. Washington, D.C.: Department of Health and Human Services, 1982. (NIH publication no 82-2453.)

10. Dohrenwend BP, Dohrenwend BS. Social status and psychological disorder: a causal inquiry. New York: Wiley-Interscience, 1969.

11. Dohrenwend BP, Dohrenwend BS, Gould MS, Link B, Neugebauer R, Wunch-Hitzig R. Mental illness in the United States: epidemiological estimates. New York: Praeger, 1980.

12. Veroff J, Kulka R, Douvan E. Mental health in America: patterns of help-seeking from 1957–1976. New York: Basic Books, 1981.

13. Kay D, Bergmann K. Epidemiology of mental disorders among the aged in the community. In: Birren J, Sloan RB, eds. Handbook of mental health and aging. Englewood Cliffs, N.J.: Prentice Hall, 1980:34–56.

14. Lee P, Lipton HL. The role of drugs and the U.S. pharmaceutical industry in health care. In: Goldberg T, ed. Review, discussion and implications of state drug substitution laws, forthcoming.

15. Schaie WW. Intelligence and problem solving. In: Biren, Sloan. op cit.:262–284.

16. Riley M, Hess B, Bond K, eds. Aging in society: selected reviews of recent research. Hillsdale, N.J.: Lawrence Erlbaum Associates, 1983.

17. Wing JK. Reasoning about madness. Oxford: Oxford U Press, 1978.

18. Mechanic D. Illness behavior, social adaptation, and the management of illness: a comparison of educational and medical models. J Nerv Ment Dis. 1977; 165:79–87.

19. Mechanic D. Disease, mortality, and the promotion of health. Health Aff. 1982; 3:28–32.

20. Dohrenwend BS, Dohrenwend BP, eds. Stressful life events and their contexts. New Brunswick, N.J.: Rutgers U Press, 1981.

21. Mechanic D. Medical sociology, 2d ed. New York: Free Press, 1978.

22. Fuchs V. "Though much is taken"—reflections on aging, health and medical care. Health Soc. 1984; 62:143–166.

23. Steering Committee on the Chronically Mentally Ill. Toward a National Plan for the Chronically Mentally Ill. Washington, D.C.: Department of Health and Human Services, 1980.

24. Goldman H, Gattozzi A, Taube C. Defining and counting the chronically mentally ill. Hosp Commun Psych. 1981; 32:21–27.

25. Stotsky BA. The nursing home and the aged psychiatric patient. New York: Appleton-Century-Crofts, 1970.

26. Gillick M. Is the care of the chronically ill a medical prerogative? N Engl J Med. 1984; 310:190–193.

27. Estes C. Social Security: the social construction of a crisis. Health Soc. 1983; 61:445–472.

28. Ball R. The financial condition of the social security program. New York: Study Group on Social Security, 1982.

――11――

Distress and Coping in Late Adolescence:
Epidemiology, Help-Seeking, and Social Adaptation

WHILE COLLEGE-AGE YOUNGSTERS report high levels of distress, such discomfort reflects to a substantial degree biological and social maturation, the uncertainties of the college environment, and evolving dilemmas in personal identity. The academic and social challenges of college encourage both anticipatory anxiety and self-conscious social comparisons often resulting in negative or insecure self-assessments. Much such discomfort is inevitable but transitory; clinicians and counselors must be careful not to put undue emphasis on such complaints or reinforce dysfunctional psychological responses.

The position I put forward here is derived from a wide variety of research efforts in social psychology. It also evolved from several studies of students I have carried out, the first of which involved all freshmen men at Stanford University and focused on perceived stress, illness behavior, and use of the Stanford Health Service over the course of the freshman year.[1] The second, on psychological distress and help-seeking, focused on a random sample of 1,502 students attending the University of Wisconsin in Madison, as well as on 156 students seeking help for personal problems at the University Psychiatric Outpatient Service and 58 students seeking help at the Counseling Center.[2,3] While the entire sample was studied cross-sectionally, freshmen and sophomores were followed prospectively as well. The third study, on health and illness behavior, involved 350 grade school children who were followed up 16 years later as young adults.[4] The final study was an intensive qualitative prospective investigation of 23 doctoral students as they anticipated, prepared for, and then took their preliminary doctoral examinations.[5] While many of the findings have been replicated in studies of adult populations, my focus is primarily on college-age youth.

The Epidemiology of Distress Among College Students

Colleges and universities vary in their admission standards but, in general, students are selected from the total population of youth on the basis of academic capacity, past performance, and coping ability. While college youth may not be unusually stable, it is plausible to assume that they have no more pathology than the population of similar age as a whole. Yet college students report high rates of psychological distress as compared with both adult populations and a representative sample of all youth within a similar age range.[2] A substantial percentage of students score in the same range on psychological distress as the average psychiatric patient. To illustrate, at Wisconsin, 20 percent of male students and 35 per cent of women students have felt that they were going to have a nervous breakdown; 6 per cent and 14 percent respectively reported this problem as somewhat or very serious. Thirty-three per cent of men and 45 per cent of women reported that they have had periods of days, weeks, or months when they couldn't take care of things because they couldn't get going. Approximately one-tenth of students defined this problem as serious.

Such crude items obviously have different meaning for varying respondents, and persons in different social contexts do not use the same comparison points. The high rates of distress reported are most reasonably seen as reflecting the situational stresses of college life, but they are not insignificant. More than one-fifth of the students in our random sample, for example, indicated that they were considerably bothered by the problems they reported, and 11 per cent indicated that these problems often prevented them from doing the things whey would like to do. Students reporting high levels of depression and anxiety were also likely to report problems in all areas of general concern to student-adolescents, including problems with parents, the student role (involving both ability and interest), career choice and their future, religious beliefs, and finances.[6] In brief, much of the anxiety and depression of these students is focused in areas of identity formation.

Seeking Help

In the study of Stanford freshman our concern was how stress affected rates of use of the Stanford Health Service over the course of the freshman year. Students, of course, adapt to stress in many ways, but I anticipated that more troubled students would come to the health service more frequently, often using common physical complaints as justification for the visit. Use of health services depends on learned patterns of illness behavior as well as on stress, and thus it was necessary to measure both variables. In the Stanford sample we found that among students inclined to depend on medical services as measured hypothetically, stress was a significant factor leading to a medical visit. The relationship was less apparent among those students less dependent on using medical services. While 73 per cent of students with a high inclination to use health services and high stress made three or more visits during the year, only 30 per cent of those with low inclination to use medical services and low stress did so.

The Wisconsin study provided a more comprehensive and rigorous context for examining help-seeking patterns among students. Here we studied not only those seeking general medical care but also psychiatric services, college counseling, religious counseling, and assistance from other formal sources of assistance, including drug information centers, a telephone suicide prevention center, a women's counseling service, faculty and administrators, and so on. Most students, at one time or another, sought informal assistance from friends and family members. A significant number also sought formal assistance. Compared with students in the random sample, students with many problems and with high levels of distress were found most commonly in the samples seeking psychiatric assistance, general counseling, and religious counseling. There is a great deal of overlap in the types of problems seen in these settings, and those seeking psychiatric care do not have fundamentally different problems than

those seeing other types of help-givers. The one exception is that
students with severe symptoms disproportionately seek or are referred to psychiatric assistance. Students seeking varying types of
help for comparable problems differ substantially in social and cultural orientations.

Controlling for symptom levels and type of symptoms, we found
considerable social selection into varying types of services depending
on the students' sociocultural characteristics, attitudes, knowledge,
and reference group orientations. If one simply compares students
with particular types of problems who either seek or do not seek care
from any source, there are few major differences. Those seeking help,
however, are more likely to know other users of services and are
more oriented to introspectiveness. But they are not very different
from the student population in social background or attitudes.

Sociocultural and attitudinal factors play a major role in the type
of help students choose.[7,8] They generally select sources of help consistent with their social background and cultural orientations, and
such factors explain where students make contact more than the type
or quality of symptoms they experience.[3] Women are disproportionately attracted to psychiatric counseling and general medical services.
Psychiatry also attracts a disproportionate number of Jewish students, and those with no religious affiliation and little religious activity. Student clients of psychiatry proportionately come from the
Northeast, have parents of Eastern European ancestry, have fathers
with high educational achievement and occupational status, and are
more likely to be majoring in the humanities, social sciences, and
fine arts. Clients of student counseling, in contrast to the population
from which they come, are younger, earlier in their educational progress, and less likely to be married. It is hardly surprising that religious counseling is more commonly used by Catholic students, those
who are religiously involved, and students oriented to traditional student culture. Psychiatry, of all sources of assistance, elicits the most
marked sociocultural selectivity.

Determinants of Distress in Late Adolescence

A simple descriptive analysis of determinants of distress is of limited
value since many of the variables of interest are interrelated, and
causal patterns are difficult to identify in the absence of a theoretical

frame of reference. Thus, after a brief review of some correlates of distress among students, my focus will be on exploring a particular perspective concerning student development.

Distress is most likely when students have difficulties in the major areas of functioning in their lives: studying and adequate school performance; social life and dating; relationship with parents; and resolution of identity in respect to future goals. The personality and coping resources students bring to college affect in large part how they approach and attempt to resolve these issues[9,11] and, thus, it remains unclear what is cause and what is effect. In our study of Wisconsin students, we carried out a variety of regression analyses to examine what personal and social characteristics made students more susceptible or immune to distress.[2] Consistent with most other studies, women report more distress than men, and younger students in each college year report more distress than those who are older. Having more close friends had a small protective effect, and a high sense of efficacy and control over one's life was associated with low distress. Students who were more oriented to introspective friends and an introspective subculture, and those who reported that they had more friends with emotional problems, were more likely to report high levels of distress. Students with high distress, as one might anticipate, also reported higher use of psychoactive drugs, alcohol, marijuana, and LSD. While these findings are suggestive, they are at best crude descriptive indicators of a complex social process.

The level of distress experienced by the majority of late adolescents reflects, I believe, their successes or failures in resolving the role demands and identity issues characteristic of their age on the one hand, and their attentiveness to their feelings and inadequacies as reflected in a high level of introspectiveness on the other. These characteristics are interrelated; problems and failures naturally draw attention to identity concerns and insecurities. But the self-consciousness characteristic of introspective youth is also culturally conditioned and may receive considerable reinforcement by some college peer groups, the subculture of the college living unit, some areas of academic study, and certain social activities on campus.

At one extreme are those students who belong to a social circle[12] of students oriented to psychodynamic psychotherapies; who spend long sessions together sharing their problems; who tend to major in the fine arts, the humanities, and the social sciences; and who are drawn to foreign movies, introspective literature, and experimentation in life styles. In sharp contrast are the more vocationally or goal-directed youth, often majoring in engineering, physical science, and business; who enthusiastically follow football; like to drink beer on weekends; identify with more conventional values; and participate in mainstream college activities. While these contrasts are a caricature, they depict a selection process that goes on within any large university in which students sort themselves on personal predispositions, social orientations, and future aspirations. To some degree, such selection takes place before college with college choices reflecting predispositions. But universities are very heterogeneous, and considerable subculture formation takes place within each institution. These subcultures, like family groups, may serve to direct or deflect attention from oneself. Such subcultures are also to some degree sex-linked, helping to explain in part both the inclination among women to report distress and their greater willingness to use varying sources of psychological assistance on campus.

Influences that direct students' attention to themselves are likely to increase the intensity and magnitude of distress they feel. A variety of studies show that attention to inner states increases the potency of emotions.[13] Buss[14] and his co-workers have developed a theory of self-consciousness based on the assumption that such self-direction results in greater self-knowledge but also an intensification of affect. These assumptions have helped organize an interesting and productive program of research. In a related development, Duval and Wicklund[15,16] have experimentally demonstrated, contrary to intuition, that increased self-awareness most frequently leads to more negative self-evaluations. A variety of studies of symptom monitoring also show that increased attention is associated with greater reported morbidity.

Persons who are introspective are more likely to react strongly to changes in their environment. In a recent study we did of psychological reactions to the nuclear accident at Three Mile Island, persons high on a measure of introspectiveness were more upset, reported more physical and behavioral symptoms, and had higher levels of psychological distress than those with lower scores. Since we studied a cohort of the same individuals following the accident, and again nine months later, we also examined to what degree distress persisted over time when the initial level of distress following the accident is taken into account. Introspective persons not only were more distressed initially but were also more likely to remain upset over time relative to their initial reactions.

In 1977, I completed a 16-year follow-up of 350 children I first studied in 1961, and was successful in relocating 95 per cent of these respondents of whom 91 per cent completed detailed questionnaires concerning their experiences.[4] Introspectiveness was associated .47 with an index of depression and anxiety, and was the most important predictor of distress among the young adults studied, controlling for 1961 measures, response bias, retrospective reports about relationships with parents, and current life stresses. The findings of this study support the hypothesis that factors in the child's development that focus the child's attention to inner states, and that encourage internal monitoring, make it more likely that the young adult will be distressed in response to such difficulties as the stresses of college life or conflicts with parents.

Distress was substantially associated with various retrospective measures we used of parental negative behavior, such as yelling, shouting, insulting the child, or lack of interest in the child. The difficulty in interpreting these findings is that such reports may be distorted and may reflect the psychological state of the respondent more than actual parental behavior. Underlying the concern with parental behavior was the idea suggested by a variety of longitudinal studies that abuse and indifference of parents, often associated with parental deviant behavior, are associated with distress, low self-evaluation, and a variety of behavior disorders.[17] Such stresses damage self-esteem and confidence and also increase the need to evaluate and to make sense of such troubling experiences.

Personal Strengths and Coping

While we tend to dwell on vulnerability, the fact is that youth are extraordinarily resilient and may overcome the greatest of social and personal adversities. Children of mentally ill parents, abused youngsters, adolescents exposed to economic deprivation, family dissolution, and periods of rejection and isolation, often manage to cope and develop adequate adult personalities, and, at times, extraordinary ones. We have given too much emphasis to adversity, and too little to the personal and social factors that enhance the capacity to overcome.

In the late 1950s, when the emphasis on vulnerability was even more pronounced than now, I intensively studied a group of 23 students preparing for preliminary doctoral examinations so as to better identify how individuals deal with a major stress of great importance to their futures.[5] It quickly became apparent that these were not passive individuals simply awaiting their fates, but rather active manipulators of their environment—planning, seeking information, preparing, devising strategies, practicing, ingratiating themselves with key decision-makers, and so on. It was perfectly clear that a theory of adaptation, simply constructed on the basis of psychodynamic processes of defense, was inadequate for describing, much less explaining, what was taking place. Studies with similar perspectives have now been carried out in a variety of contexts, showing clearly the importance of active coping, not only in dealing with stressors, but in psychological growth.

Successful adaptation depends on having and exercising the skills relevant to dealing with usual and sometimes extraordinary challenges and adversities—what is generally referred to as coping. Coping, however, requires a reasonable level of attention and psychological equilibrium, and various cognitive mechanisms— usually referred to as defenses—make possible control over anxiety, depression, and fear. Also, the willingness to become engaged, and to confront the possibility of failure, requires motivation. Without the energy of incentive there is no stress, nor is there growth. Social organization provides the motivation through incentives that reward those who meet and exceed standard expectations. Family ties and friendship frequently provide incentives but also social supports that facilitate defenses and help control self-doubt and other negative feelings. Coping effectiveness, of course, depends on how successfully we teach youth to face prospective challenges and adversity, and schooling is only a limited aspect of this larger picture.

If our focus is less on youth with various disorders and more on those who are competent and well-adjusted, it is clear that they are active, purposeful actors who anticipate future challenges relative to aspirations and goals, who plan their agendas more or less carefully, who rehearse problems and alternative solutions, who seek information from peers, parents, and other sources, who pace themselves in approaching new situations, and so on. As Silber and his colleagues put it; "The active search for manageable levels of challenge in newness is more characteristic of the coping behavior of competent adolescents than a stabilized adaptation to the environment with maximal reduction of tension" (p. 265).[9]

The typical adolescent's approach to college studies is an example to some extent of the adaptive strategies of most youngsters. Except for the very exceptional, college students, while aspiring to do well, usually feel that it is unrealistic to conform to all the expectations they face in the variety of courses they take. Since most students measure their learning and progress by the grades they earn, they quickly focus on the material on which they will be tested, giving less attention to other aspects of their course work. While faculty may be emphasizing broad issues, the student commonly feels the urgency of "making the grade."[18] In this respect, students learn a broad range of strategies to juggle the competing demands in their lives. They give disproportionate time to the more demanding courses; they counterbalance difficult courses with "gut" courses; they take courses on a pass-fail basis, which often means doing as little as possible; and they quickly "psych out" what is relevant for examinations. This emphasis on separating what will be tested from the broad educational concerns of any program has been found to be major organizing themes for students in undergraduate education,[18] professional schools,[19] medical schools,[20] and in graduate programs.[21,5] It isn't that students are cynical—relatively few are. Their stance reflects the need to make the challenges faced more certain and manageable, and managing their anxieties.

Research studies are now providing support for the views of many thoughtful observers that adolescents require a challenging environment that facilitates the development of adaptive skills. Through active engagement with responsibility, young people learn the skills necessary for most adult roles and develop a sense of efficacy and self-esteem as they witness their own growth and maturity. Elder[22] studied a cohort of children born in 1920–1921, who grew up during the Great Depression. Data were available on anxiety and tension, psychosomatic illnesses, behavior disorders, serious somatic illnesses, and psychotic reactions in adulthood. Children from the working class faced greater adversities during the depression and had more problems later. But middle-class children who faced deprivation were more symptom-free in adulthood than those who had been sheltered. Twenty-six per cent of the nondeprived middleclass had behavior disorder problems in contrast to 7 per cent in the deprived group. Heavy drinking in adulthood was much more common in the nondeprived middle class (43 per cent versus 24 per cent). The study cannot provide much indication of the dynamics here, but deprivation may demand more responsibility and assistance from the adolescent, which not only contributes to the family but to the adolescent's self-respect and future adaptive capacities.

Seligman[23] has argued that exposure to difficulties is important not only for successful development but also for a sense of efficacy that protects against depression. He believes that many current problems may stem from removing challenge during important developmental stages and making things too easy. As he puts it: "A sense of worth, mastery, or self-esteem cannot be bestowed. It can only be earned. If it is given away, it ceases to be worth having, and it ceases to contribute to individual dignity. If we remove the obstacles, difficulties, anxiety, and competition from the lives of our young people, we may no longer see generations of young people who have a sense of dignity, power and worth" (p. 159).

While affluence used wastefully is often the focus of concern of critics, most studies suggest that affluence contributes positively to effective performance, health outcomes, and psychological well-being. It does so, I believe, because it provides opportunities for developing skills in more academically oriented and more demanding schools and in a wide array of extracurricular activities. Youngsters develop skills and self-esteem not only in jobs, but also in musical and artistic performances, in theatrical groups, in team sports, in purposeful clubs, in pursuing skill-demanding hobbies, and so on.

One thing is clear: adaptive capacities do not thrive in passive environments that make no demands, require no special efforts, and yield no sense of accomplishment. Studies showing the enormous amounts of time youngsters spend watching television may point to a serious impediment to effective development in some children. Television, like any other technology, may be used in various ways, and may actively engage the imagination. But, too often, it is an escape from activity and responsibility, a means of filling time without many benefits.

A great deal of attention has been devoted to the effects of television violence on children, but the passivity among chronic viewers, and television's use as an escape from engaging the environment, may in the long run be more serious consequences. Although the work is limited, there are some studies suggesting that longer viewing is related to depressive affect in youngsters,[24] and more intelligent youth watch less violence.[25] Cause and effect here are difficult to separate. It may be that more unhappy, insecure, and isolated youngsters watch television to escape their difficulties and frustrations.

Implications for Student Services

Students experiment broadly with varying life-styles and roles and it is easy to give undue significance to particular patterns of behavior that seem inappropriate. Most problems among college students, however, are self-limited, reflecting both the ambiguities and wide latitude of the student role and the identity issues late adolescents typically encounter. Many students of college age are eager to discuss their problems and relatively receptive to using available services. They often overestimate the significance of the problems and troubles they face and tend to regard them as more unique than they really are. It is clear that many of the students seen at student psychiatry, student health, and other helping agencies on campus have problems that are shared by numerous other students, most of whom do not seek special assistance.

Students facing rather ordinary problems of late adolescence often receive intrapsychic counseling that may reinforce their already high levels of introspectiveness, which, as I noted earlier, heightens the sense of discomfort and also makes it more likely that students will seek assistance. Thus, students typically seen in student psychiatry and other types of counseling situations are already relatively high in the inclination to give attention to their feelings.

In many instances, counseling that focuses on clarifying objectives and developing ways of achieving them is more appropriate than intrapsychic interventions. Many students, facing the typical crises of adolescent identity, do better by setting tangible goals and working toward their achievement than by focusing on themselves. Student life is extraordinarily diffuse with few clear expectations beyond adequate academic performance. Defining and achieving clear objectives is extraordinarily reinforcing for young people, and a source of confidence and self-esteem. Often, what students need most is help in devising a strategy to move toward defining and achieving objectives.

In sum, for the typical adolescent in crisis, much of the assistance necessary involves coping more than psychological defense. Students typically have a difficult time deciding on objectives or knowing how they can achieve those they define. Not infrequently, the difficulty in making plans, and lack of structure characteristic of the college environment, captures the student in a cycle of inactivity, boredom, and decreased self-esteem.

The challenge, therefore, is to facilitate adaptive skills not by making students patients but by enhancing their ability to clarify goals, to plan, to make decisions, to devise strategies and to resolve problems. This can often be facilitated by support and encouragement and by guiding a better appreciation of the extent to which the issues of concern are widely shared by others of the same age. Information on how others have successfully managed comparable problems may be particularly helpful. Peer groups are extraordinarily influential during late adolescence, and peers can be used quite effectively to teach and rehearse solutions that they have successfully used. Finally, providing effective assistance requires knowing the campus environment, its subcultures and living groups. Problems are sometimes reduced by achieving a better fit between the values and aspirations of the student and the dominant ethos of his/her living group.

References

1. Mechanic D, Volkart E. Stress, illness behavior and the sick role. Amer Soc Rev. 1961; 26:51–58.
2. Mechanic D, Greenley J. The prevalence of psychological distress and help seeking in a college student population. Soc Psych. 1976; 11:1–14.
3. Greenley J, Mechanic D. Social selection in seeking help for psychological problems. J Health Soc Behav. 1976; 17:249–262.
4. Mechanic D. Development of psychological distress among young adults. Arch Gen Psych. 1979; 36:1233–1239.
5. Mechanic D. Students under stress: a study in the social psychology of adaptation. Madison: U of Wisconsin Press, 1978.
6. Newmann J. Sex differences in life problems and psychological distress. M.A. thesis, Madison: U of Wisconsin, 1975.
7. Linn LS. Social characteristics and social interaction in the utilization of a psychiatric outpatient clinic. J Health Soc Behav. 1967; 8:3–14.
8. Scheff TJ. Users and non-users of a student psychiatric clinic. J Health Human Behav. 1966; 7:114–121.
9. Silber E, Hamburg DA, Coelho GV, Murphey EB, Rosenberg R, Pearlin L. Adaptive behavior in competent adolescents. Arch Gen Psych. 1961; 5:354–365.
10. Silber E, et al. Competent adolescents coping with college decisions. Arch Gen Psych. 1961; 5:517–527.

11. Coelho GV, Hamburg DA, Murphey EB. Coping strategies in a new learning environment. Arch Gen Psych. 1963; 9:433–443.

12. Kadushin C. Why people go to psychiatrists. New York: Atherton, 1969.

13. Mechanic D. Adolescent health and illness behavior: hypotheses for the study of distress in youth. J Human Stress. 1983; 9:4–13.

14. Buss AH. Self-consciousness and social anxiety. San Francisco: WH Freeman, 1980.

15. Duval S, Wicklund RA. A theory of objective self-awareness. New York: Academic Press, 1972.

16. Wicklund RA. Objective self-awreness. In: Berkowitz L, ed. Advances in experimental social psychology, vol. 8. New York: Academic Press, 1975.

17. Robins LN. Follow-up studies of behavior disorders in children. In: Quay HG, Werry JS, eds. Psychopathological disorders of childhood, 2d ed. New York: John Wiley and Sons, 1979.

18. Becker HS, Geer B, Hughes EC, Strauss AL. Boys in white: student culture in medical school. Chicago: U of Chicago Press, 1961.

19. Becker HS, et al. Making the grade: the academic side of college life. New York: John Wiley and Sons, 1968.

20. Orth CD, III. Social structure and learning climate: the first year at the Harvard Business School. Boston. Harvard Graduate School of Business Administration, 1963.

21. Sanford M. Making it in graduate school. Berkeley, Calif.: Montaigne, 1976.

22. Elder GH, Jr. Children of the Great Depression: social change in life experience. Chicago: U of Chicago Press, 1974.

23. Seligman MEP. Helplessness: on depression, development and death. San Francisco: WH Freeman, 1975.

24. Lefkowitz M, Huesmann LR. Concomitants of television violence viewing in children. In: Palmer EL, Door A, eds. Children and the faces of television: teaching, violence, selling. New York: Academic Press, 1980:163–181.

25. Dorr A, Kovaric P. Some of the people some of the time—but which people? Televised violence and its effects. In: Palmer, Dorr, eds. op cit.: 183–199.

26. Gerbner G, Gross L. The violent face of television and its lessons. In: Palmer, Dorr, eds. op cit.: 154.

Mental Health and Social Policy:

Some Needed Initiatives for the 1980s

MENTAL DISORDERS are a major source of suffering and disability, cause havoc in families and the community, and account for a large load on medical care institutions, social agencies, and sheltered facilities. In 1980, mental illness was the third most expensive class of disorders accounting for more than $20 billion of health care expenditures.[1] Only the circulatory disorders—including heart disease, stroke, hypertension—and all disorders of the digestive system were more costly in the aggregate. Moreover, much of medical care utilization associated with mental disorder is not included in the above calculations since many of these problems are expressed somatically or are associated with disorders classified under a variety of other diagnostic entities.

Problems of depression, phobias, and substance abuse are most common,[2] but the image of mental illness in the public mind is shaped most substantially by the highly visible chronically mentally ill who suffer from significant impairments, compose a large part of the homeless, and are often upsetting or even frightening to the public who encounter them. While the population of chronically mentally ill is estimated to be no more than 1 per cent of the total population,[3] these persons constitute an enormous burden on the community and a serious challenge to social policy.

A variety of forces dramatically reshaped the mental health services system and the location of care in the past 30 years. These included: the growing burden on state mental health budgets of institutionalizing the chronically mentally ill; the widespread use of psychotropic drugs that alleviated some of the most troublesome symptoms of schizophrenic patients; the professional attack on the large public mental hospital and its role in the development of secondary disabilities associated with institutional tenure; and a vigorous civil liberties movement on behalf of the rights of the mentally ill.[4] These influences encouraged the release of many long-term patients from public mental hospitals and shorter periods of stay for newly admitted patients. But most chronic mental patients are highly disabled and unable to support themselves. The introduction of Medicare and Medicaid in 1966 and the growth of Social Security Disability Insurance and Supplemental Security Income allowed the retention of patients in community settings or alternative institutions such as nursing homes that expanded rapidly with federal support.

The major thrust in deinstitutionalization did not occur until the mid-1960s, when these welfare programs were first initiated or expanded. From 1955 to 1965, inpatient populations of the mentally ill showed an average annual decrease of 1.5 per cent. Between 1965 and 1980, the average was more than 6 per cent per year.[5] Federal programs allowed states to shift part of their mounting financial burden for chronic care to the federal government by moving patients from state institutions. The number of mental patients in public hospitals were reduced from their peak of 560,000 in 1955 to approximately 125,000 at present. But three-quarters of a million elderly and other chronic patients, having either a primary or secondary mental illness diagnosis, are now housed in nursing homes.[3]

It is widely appreciated that many demented elderly patients reside in nursing homes, but the significant number of younger impaired mental patients in these institutions are relatively invisible. It remains unclear whether the typical care of younger chronic patients in nursing homes even approximates the quality of care, admittedly poor, typical of many of the large state and county mental hospitals prior to deinstitutionalization. Patients in nursing homes are commonly overmedicated to ease management and spend much of their time doing nothing. It has been repeatedly demonstrated, however, that inactivity is extraordinarily harmful, typically resulting in additional disabilities and poor functioning.

The numbers of patients resident in mental hospitals and total hospital days for psychiatric care has significantly declined in the United States from 168 million days in 1969 to 95 million days in 1978,[6] but the number of admissions to psychiatric beds has substantially increased, with a large growth of admissions in the general hospital sector. Inpatient days for psychiatric care in general hospitals approximately doubled between 1969 and 1978, increasing from approximately 1 per cent of total psychiatric days in 1969 to one-fifth of the total in 1978.

The aggregate data on hospital days combine two very different populations, the insured and the noninsured. Those having insurance commonly receive their care in general hospitals and increasingly in private psychiatric beds, the fastest-growing component of inpatient psychiatric care. Average length of stay is relatively brief and costs are comparable to other medical sectors. Patients without insurance, or those who have exhausted coverage, are invariably referred to public institutions who retain only the most seriously impaired. Other chronics are returned to community settings as soon as feasible, often without necessary services or adequate follow-up. Many of these patients suffer from repeated exacerbations of their disorders, have multiple rehospitalizations, and commonly shuttle between the public mental health system and the correctional system. They may live with family members, in supervised settings, or in private housing, or move among these alternatives depending on availability, their clinical status, and their success in maintaining relationships with others. Many refuse psychiatric care and cannot be hospitalized as a consequence of the stricter criteria for civil commitment that now prevail. Increasing numbers of chronics appear to be homeless although reliable information is difficult to obtain.

The above oversimplifies trends given our decentralized system, variations among community health services systems, the varying diagnoses and personal histories of patients and economic conditions, and medical and social welfare entitlements that differ from one community to another. Patterns of care also depend on the culture of ethnic enclaves in which the mentally ill are embedded, patients' definitions of the nature of mental illness and the psychiatric system, and community tolerance and understanding. Professionals in touch with young chronics report that a growing number of these patients are aggressive, have antipsychiatric ideologies, and are demanding and uncooperative.[7,8] Whether there is a significant change in the composition of the younger chronic group as compared with earlier cohorts, or whether a subgroup of particularly difficult patients in community settings influence the perception of such patients overall, remains unclear. Whatever the specific reality, and it may differ significantly in large urban areas, the fact remains that many chronic mental patients pose formidable problems of care, rehabilitation, and social control that require vigorous and effectively coordinated programs that have medical, psychosocial, and educational dimensions. Such programs exist as isolated models but have not been widely adopted.

Much of the difficulty is in the intractable nature of schizophrenia and the vigorous and sustained efforts necessary for relatively modest achievements with these patients. But providing appropriate services has been very much complicated by the fragmentation of funding, the unintended but perverse effects of health legislation and regulations primarily developed with other disabled populations in mind, and cost-shifting among varying levels of government. Despite the enormity of mental health policy issues, there is no clearly defined arena or forum for bringing coherence to the wide array of facilities and funding streams that impact the welfare of chronic patients.

As compared with other disease-oriented interest groups, the mentally ill, and particularly chronic patients, are significantly disadvantaged in the political processes affecting the composition of health budgets and other programs relevant to the sustained research, demonstration, and practice efforts necessary. These difficulties include:

1. The mentally ill, particularly those suffering from psychiatric and other chronic and severe disorders, lack the skills, capacities, and social standing to effectively represent their own interests in the public arena.
2. Mental illness retains considerable social stigma in comparison to other disease categories, which deters influential former patients, patients, and families from engaging in "personal public advocacy."
3. There is much fragmentation and lack of cooperation among voluntary groups representing subsets of the mentally ill in

the public arena due in part to contrasting philosophies and varying definitions of the problem. Thus, advocates of the mentally ill, alcoholics, substance abusers, and the developmentally disabled almost never form a united front.

4. Both public and private insurance treat mental illness benefits different from other disorders in terms of coverage, maximum benefits, co-insurance, and deductibles. This reflects historic conceptions of the special nature of mental illness and apprehension about costs. Such practices reinforce existing prejudices.

5. The subspecialty of psychiatry and other mental health professions do not stand high among influentials in the health arena.

6. Mentally ill patients are commonly blamed for their plight and the diagnosis of mental illness often results in attributions that challenge the capacity of the mentally ill to function reliably or make sound judgments in areas unrelated to their illnesses.

7. Much of the financial support for the treatment and rehabilitation of the mentally ill is embedded in medical insurance and federal entitlement programs conceptualized and organized in terms of illnesses and disabilities of a nonpsychiatric kind. Administrative procedures and decisions are often prejudicial or detrimental to persons with chronic psychiatric conditions.

8. Policymakers and administrators responsible for major programs affecting the mentally ill, such as Medicare and Medicaid, are often inadequately informed about the special character of mental illness and the unique needs of these patients.

Needed Initiatives

Residence patterns for the chronic patient have shifted dramatically, but most state funding continues to be concentrated in public mental hospitals that serve only a minority of this disadvantaged population. There is little doubt that the reduction of hospital patient populations has facilitated more and better inpatient care for those who remain, transforming many custodial institutions into active treatment settings. But there remains a significant imbalance between expenditures for inpatients and many patients who in earlier periods would have been confined to public institutions and who clearly need assistance despite their outpatient status. While part of the problem is surely the underfinancing of care for the chronically mentally ill, significant resistance to closing redundant institutions and moving funds to community care comes from employees, unions, and communities for whom mental hospitals provide an important economic base.

There has been much merit in the conversion of custodial institutions to more active treatment contexts and no one seeks to lose these gains. There is also impressive evidence that most chronic mental patients, among whom schizophrenics constitute a majority, can do relatively well with appropriate care that monitors medical need and promotes social functioning in the community at a cost comparable to or less than present patterns of care that lack coherent organization. Achievement of a more coordinated and effective pattern of care will require redirection of reimbursement patterns so as to allow appropriate choices and trade-offs between traditional medical and hospital services and more broad sociomedical services in community contexts. Given the realities of funding constraints, it becomes even more essential to make cost-effective decisions on behalf of the chronic population.

Experimental and Other Innovative Demonstrations

Planning for care of the chronically mentally ill has not suffered for lack of innovative programmatic ideas. Careful experimental evaluation has been less common and little effort has been made to facilitate transferring successful programs or their components from one context to another given the complexity of organizational arrangements, financing, and professionals' definitions of their appropriate roles.

An early community care experiment in California by Fairweather and his colleagues[9] established a community group living situation for chronic posthospital patients that included the organization of a janitorial service. As compared with traditional hospital care, patients in the program had greater work productivity and less psychosocial maladjustment, and even during periods of maximum supervision, the experimental program was less expensive than customary services. The experiment was a success, but the program was not widely adopted. As Fairweather saw it:

> The reason clearly was that to accept it demanded rather extensive social role and status changes among professional people. They had to become problem solvers and had in fact, in the final analysis, to become consultants rather than supervisors and, indirectly, to phase themselves out of the patients' society in order to give first-class citizenship to ex-mental patients. It was this role that was so difficult for professionals to accept.[10]

Other innovative community service programs have been developed in which hospitalization is avoided and problems are dealt with through home visits and systems intervention. During periods of crisis, or when no adequate permanent home is available, patients are placed in carefully selected "foster families" supported by clinical supervision, instruction of caretakers, and clinical home visits.[11] Families taking such patients receive a daily payment for room, board, and client care. Other programs train and use community members to assist chronic patients in daily life activities. Some communities have established patient apartment complexes, clubs and recreation centers, and a variety of sheltered work situations for the chronically disabled.[12]

One important experiment in Wisconsin involved a training program in community living for chronic patients.[13,14] This study compared an educational coping model with a progressive hospital care unit. An unselected group of patients referred for admission to a mental hospital was randomly assigned to experimental and control groups. The control group received good hospital treatment, linked with a progressive program of community aftercare services. The experimental group was assisted in developing an independent living situation in the community, given social support, and taught simple living skills, such as budgeting, job seeking, and use of public transportation. Patients in both groups were evaluated at various intervals by independent researchers. The findings showed that it was possible for highly impaired patients to be cared for almost exclusively in the community. Compared with control patients, patients in the experimental group made a more adequate community adjustment as measured by higher earnings from work, involvement in more social activities, more contact with friends, and more satisfaction with their life situation. Experimental patients at follow-up had fewer symptoms than the controls. This experiment illustrated that a logically organized and aggressive community program can effectively manage even highly impaired patients in the community, with minimal use of hospitals.

Such successful community programs are not without costs. A careful economic cost-benefit analysis of the above experiment, taking into account a wide range of hidden as well as explicit costs, such as welfare payments and supervised residency costs, suggests that while such programs yield a net benefit, they are not necessarily *less expensive* in economic terms than more conventional approaches.[15] Moreover, there are social costs in maintaining patients in the community, as compared with hospital care during the more acute phases of disorder, as measured by law violations and assaultive behavior. The prevalence of such behavior was low, but not inconsequential. We still need careful study of the best mix of community care and short-term and prudent use of hospital facilities. Gudeman and Shore,[16] on the basis of their experiences at the Massachusetts Mental Health Center, estimate that 6 per cent of their chronic population, such as assaultive and highly disruptive patients, would be better served in specialized facilities than in the community. Projected to the population of Massachusetts, this would require 861 psychiatric beds. While proponents and opponents of mental hospital care may argue about appropriate criteria, it seems apparent that some small component of the chronic population would be better cared for in an appropriate but humane institution.

The visibility of the homeless in large cities, many who are chronic mental patients, focuses disproportionate attention on a group that apparently has no or very limited family supports. In contrast, many chronic mental patients continue to live in family settings or relate to relatives actively involved with their welfare. Much is gained by supporting natural groups when they are available and assisting them to cope with the problems and burdens of caring for a seriously impaired relative. Fortunately, there have been some exciting developments in understanding better how to assist family members to cope successfully with a schizophrenic patient.

As early as 1962, Brown and his associates in London reported that schizophrenic patients with relatives who showed high expressed emotion in a family interview deteriorated more frequently than patients living in a low emotional involvement environment.[17] This observation was replicated in a variety of research settings in various countries. Emotional involvement in the case of schizophrenic patients largely denotes excessive involvement, negative emotions, and criticisms. While the effects on the patients' symptoms are attenuated to a considerable degree when patients are maintained on psychotropic medications, emotional involvement affects medicated patients as well. It seems that schizophrenics cannot tolerate high levels of stress, and psychotropic drugs in part blunt the effects of stress. Patients who have less face-to-face contact with overinvolved relatives are also less likely to relapse.[18,19] Negative emotions of relatives is also related to family tolerance and expectations, which in turn relates to the patient's retention outside the hospital.[20]

In a recent, controlled social intervention trial in London, schizophrenic patients having intense contact with relatives demonstrating high expressed emotion were randomly assigned to either routine outpatient care or an intervention program for patients and their families emphasizing education about schizophrenia and the role of expressed emotion.[21] The intervention also included family sessions in the home and relatives' groups. All patients were maintained on psychotropic drugs. After nine months, 50 per cent of the 24 control patients relapsed but only 9 per cent in the experimental group. There were no relapses in 73 per cent of experimental families where the aims of the intervention were achieved.

A similar experimental trial was carried out in California, where family members of schizophrenics were taught about the condition, were instructed in problem-solving techniques, and efforts were made to reduce family tensions.[22,23] Follow-up at nine months found that patients in families receiving such interventions had a much lower rate of exacerbations than those in a control group receiving clinic-based individual supportive care. Only one patient in the intervention group (6 per cent) was judged to have a relapse, in contrast to eight (44 per cent) in the control group.

Long-Term Impacts

A discouraging aspect of care for chronic patients is that even the successful programs require continuing efforts over many years. Long-term studies of programs for chronic patients, whether in the hospital or the community, indicate that improvements in patient functioning and performance require persistence and continuity. Wing and Brown,[24] in a study of three British mental hospitals in the period 1960 to 1968, found that with changes in these hospitals, patients benefited in the early years, but over time some of the progress was lost. These data reflect how difficult it is to maintain progress with chronically impaired patients over long periods of time. Comparable findings characterize community care. The progress achieved by the community care program described by Stein and Test[13] was lost once the program ended and patients returned to traditional care. A five-year follow-up of the patients studied by Pasamanick and associates[25] also found deterioration of patient functioning following the termination of the experiment.[26]

These studies suggest, comparable to other studies involving interventions to change health behaviors, that while short-term improvements can be achieved, long-term progress is a more formidable goal for both patients and those responsible for their care. It is not clear to what extent initial progress is in part assisted by the hope, enthusiasm, and novelty associated with innovative efforts or new programs. The results suggest, however, the importance of renewing periodically the energies, interest, and commitment of the treatment staff. In many instances, failure results primarily from the loss of stable funding. Once we make the commitment to the need for longitudinal responsibility for chronic patients, identifying means to maintain efforts over time and insure stable funding are continuing challenges.

Appropriate Mix of Health Personnel

Psychiatry is one of the few medical specialties anticipated to be in relatively short supply in the future. In recent years we have seen less interest in psychiatry among medical students and residents, and those choosing psychiatric careers are more oriented to biological psychiatry than to community care or rehabilitiation. Few psychiatrists seem enthusiastic about working with the chronically mentally ill. Sophisticated drug management is essential for appropriate care of most psychiatric illness, and to avoid the dangers of serious side effects associated with psychotropic drugs, but psychiatrists might more realistically function in this area as consultants to practitioners organizing chronic care than as primary caretakers. There clearly seems to be an appropriate role for a new nursing specialty, the psychiatric nurse practitioner.

Psychiatric nurse practitioners can be an invaluable resource in staffing a variety of institutional facilities, outpatient services, and community care programs for the mentally ill.[27] While psychologists and social workers also have essential roles to play, the appropriately trained nurse practitioner is potentially in a strategic position. They bring to this role a long tradition in socioemotional and supportive aspects of care and some familiarity with medication monitoring and pharmacological issues. Also, nurses are increasingly conversant with behavior modification techniques and supportive group therapies. The close association between nursing and medicine insures credibility with physicians and patients in the area of medication administration and monitoring and psychiatric nurse practitioners can also serve as effective "boundary practitioners" for many patients who resist treatment within the psychiatric sector but more readily accept general medical and nursing assistance. A major problem even among chronic patients is their resistance to psychiatric conceptualizations of their distress and behavior. Nurses with enhanced mental health capabilities could play an important leadership role. Since nurse practitioners and nurse specialists have comparable roles in other areas of patient care, the necessary adjustments and role transitions would not be insurmountable.

In reality, nurses and other nonpsychiatric personnel have provided most of the available care for chronic patients. However, their formal training has not fully prepared them for the tasks they perform. The psychiatric nurse practitioner, for example, should receive more intensive training in psychopharmacology and with improved training may prescribe a limited range of psychotropic drugs using approved protocols. While this would require legislative changes, nurse practitioners in other areas already have such responsibility and authority, for example pediatric nurse practitioners. In addition, more intensive training in behavior techniques and cognitive therapies would be essential as well. Since nurses in such roles, especially in community contexts, also have major managerial responsibilities, training should include a broader understanding of the complex range of social programs and financial entitlements that are central to maintaining mental patients in the community. Such nurses, in short, must learn to be effective case managers as part of their role.

Key Policy Issues

The care of the chronic mental patient is a formidable task requiring a coordinated strategy, cooperation among varying levels of government, a clear definition of responsibility, and a longitudinal perspective and approach. Private psychiatric beds have been expanding rapidly to serve insured populations with less incapacitating disorders, but it is an illusion to anticipate that the interests of these difficult and uninsured patients will require anything less than sustained state responsibility. Even with more generous reimbursement, contractors in the private sector are likely to have little interest in these highly impaired patients. While most of the mentally ill can be managed reasonably within the context of our larger health care system, the chronic patient requires central public policy attention. It is inevitable that these patients will require special efforts by specially trained and motivated professionals functioning within a coherent and integrated system of financing and service delivery.

Chronic mental patients in community settings face formidable problems in coping, including acquisition of appropriate medical care and mental health services, housing, nutrition, recreation, and sustained social contact. These patients are repeatedly brought to emergency rooms, hospitals, and jails during periods of extreme stress and psychotic disorganization, and consume enormous medical and other community resources that are used ineffectively. While in the community, they are often isolated, neglected, and out of touch with an established system of services that is organized to respond realistically to their needs. A well-organized community program based on the care principles discussed in the review of experimental programs could prevent much needless and expensive hospitalization and imprisonment, monitor medical and mental health status more closely, and promote higher levels of functioning and activity.

Similar conceptions of community care served as the basis for the Community Support Program,[28,29] a major national plan for the chronically ill prior to the decentralization of federal mental health programs. Responsibility for these patients now almost exclusively rests with local and state authorities. A single authority at the local level funded to assume responsibility for the total array of hospital and community services for the chronic population is needed. While no fully integrated system exists including all sources of funding, Wisconsin's funding formula for mental health and social services holds counties responsible for the entire spectrum of necessary care, thus providing an incentive for careful choices among alternatives. In one county, 83 per cent of expenditures for chronic patients are in the form of community services as contrasted with hospital care.[30]

By funding an identifiable program with broad responsibilities, incentives are developed for carefully considered trade-offs between inpatient and community care alternatives. Following the logic of an HMO, such organizations have incentives to avoid unnecessary expensive care and alternatively invest these resources in building and supporting a more appropriate spectrum of community services. Such systems also induce responsibility for monitoring patients appropriately since failure to do so wastes scarce resources essential to support community services and employ appropriate professional personnel.

While the concept of county responsibility, as developed in Wisconsin, serves as an excellent beginning framework, the larger ideal would be to integrate responsibility and funding for the total array of medical, mental health, social services, and social welfare funding for this population. The multiplicity of funding authorities and sources of finance make full integration unlikely, but even partial integration of selected categorical programs, each with its own eligibility criteria and regulatory limitations, would contribute immensely to better organized and effective care. Achieving this requires complex negotiations, agreement on waivers, and considerable technical expertise. It should be possible to fund at least the medical, mental health, and social services care of chronic patients on a capitated basis, but achieving this in more than an isolated instance will require our very best and sustained efforts.

With the decentralization of mental health services, and funding complexities, a formidable problem is diffusing effective approaches from one setting to another. Barriers to replication of successful programs include resistance to redirection of reimbursement from hospital to community, required changes in professional roles and relationships, lack of local leadership, financial incentives to persist with traditional approaches, and entrenched interest groups that benefit from the current organization of services.[31]

While the political barriers are substantial, much of the problem is also evident in the poor flow of practical information, the lack of confidence many mental health professionals have in changing course, and the difficulty of gaining the administrative, managerial, organizational, and technical mental health experience that allows successful techniques to be transferred and fitted to varying local circumstances. We could do more to transfer effective approaches by bringing teams of appropriate officials and professionals to sites where they could learn directly from those involved in new programs, and to share clinical and organizational experiences. Such "teams" might include individuals having the financial, administrative, and professional authority and expertise necessary to implement their goals once they return to their own communities.

In summary, we face an extraordinary challenge in caring for the chronically mentally ill, particularly in light of cost-containment pressures on the health care system as a whole and in a context of tightening eligibility within many programs on which the chronic patient depends. It seems unlikely in this context that much new funding will become available for this population, making it even more critical that existing budgets be used wisely and to best effect. Patterns of care continue to be fragmented and poorly organized, and the range and complexity of existing entitlements requires ingenuity and energy to negotiate. The single most important contribution to patient care we could make in coming years is to consolidate funding sources at the local level allowing rational calculations and decision-making among alternatives. The trick is to get there from our present starting point.

References

1. U.S. Department of Human Services. Health—United States, 1983. Hyattsville, Md.: National Center for Health Statistics, 1983. (DHHS publication no. [PHS] 84–1232:166.)
2. Robins L, et al. Lifetime prevalence of specific psychiatric disorders in three sites. Arch Gen Psych. 1984; 41:949–958.
3. Goldman HH, Gattozzi AA, Taube CA. Defining and counting the chronically mentally ill. Hosp Commun Psych. 1981; 32:21–27.
4. Mechanic D. Mental health and social policy, 2d ed. Englewood Cliffs, N.J.: Prentice-Hall, 1980.
5. Gronfein W. Rhetoric and reality in mental health policy: the case of the state hospitals. Rutgers-Princeton Program in Mental Health Research, 1984.

6. Kiesler CA, Sibulkin AE. Proportion of inpatient days for mental disorders: 1969–1978. Hosp Commun Psych. 1983; 34:606–611.

7. Schwartz S, Goldfinger S. The new chronic patient: clinical characteristics of an emerging subgroup. Hosp Commun Psych. 1981; 32:470–474.

8. Sheets J, Prevost J, Reihman J. Young adult chronic patients: three hypothesized subgroups. Hosp Commun Psych. 1982; 33:197–202.

9. Fairweather GW, et al. Community life for the mentally ill: an alternative to institutional care. Chicago: Aldine, 1969.

10. Fairweather G. The development, evaluation, and diffusion of rehabilitative programs: a social change process. In: Stein LI, Test MA, eds. Alternatives to mental hospital treatment. New York: Plenum, 1978.

11. Polak P. A comprehensive system of alternatives to psychiatric hospitalization. In Stein LI, Test MA. eds. op cit.:115–137.

12. Stein LI, Test MA, eds. op cit.

13. Stein LI, Test MA. Alternatives to mental hospital treatment I. Conceptual model, treatment program and clinical evaluation. Arch Gen Psych. 1980; 37:392–397.

14. Stein LI, Test MA. Alternatives to mental hospital treatment III. Social cost. Arch Gen Psych. 1980; 37:409–412.

15. Weisbrod BA, Test MA, Stein LI. Alternatives to mental hospital treatment II. Economic benefit-cost analysis. Arch Gen Psych. 1980; 37:400–405.

16. Gudeman JE, Shore MF. Beyond deinstitutionalization: a new class of facilities for the mentally ill. N Engl J Med. 1984; 311:832–836.

17. Brown GW, Birley JLT, Wing JK. Influence of family life on the course of schizophrenic disorders: a replication. Brit J Psych. 1972; 121:241–258.

18. Vaughn CE, Leff JP. The influence of family and social factors on the course of psychiatric illness: a comparison of schizophrenic and depressed neurotic patients. Brit J Psych. 1976; 129:125–137.

19. Leff J. Social and psychological causes of acute attack. In: Wing JK. ed. Schizophrenia: toward a new synthesis. New York: Grune and Stratton, 1978:139–165.

20. Greenley JR. The psychiatric patient's family and length of hospitalization. J Health Soc Behav. 1972; 13:25–37.

21. Leff J, et al. A controlled trial of social intervention in the families of schizophrenic patients. Brit J Psych. 1982; 141:121–134.

22. Falloon IRH, Boyd J, McGill C. Family care of schizophrenia. New York: Guilford Press, 1984.

23. Falloon IRH, et al. Family management in the prevention of exacerbations of schizophrenia: a controlled study. N Engl J Med. 1982; 306:1437–1440.
24. Wing JK, Brown GW. Institutionalism and schizophrenia: a comparative study of three mental hospitals, 1960–1968. Cambridge, England: Cambridge U Press, 1970.
25. Pasamanick B, Scarpitti FR, Dinitz FR. Schizophrenics in the community: an experimental study in the prevention of hospitalization. New York: Appleton-Century-Crofts, 1967.
26. Davis A, Pasamanick B, Dinitz S. Schizophrenics in the new custodial community: five years after the experiment. Columbus: Ohio State U, 1974.
27. Mechanic D. Nursing and mental health care: expanding future possibilities for nursing services. In: Aiken L, ed. Nursing in the 1980s—crises, opportunities, challenges. Philadelphia: Lippincott, 1982:343–358.
28. Turner J, Tenhoor WJ. The NIMH community support program: pilot approach to a needed social reform. Schiz Bull. 1978; 4:319–344.
29. National Institute of Mental Health. A network for caring: the community support program of the National Institute of Mental Health. Washington, D.C.: Department of Health and Human Services, 1982. (DHHS publication no. [ADM] 81–106.)
30. Stein LI, Ganser LJ. Wisconsin system for funding mental health services. In: Talbott J, ed. New directions for mental health services: unified mental health system. San Francisco: Jossey-Bass, 1983:25–32.
31. Mechanic D. Future issues in health care: social policy and the rationing of medical services. New York: Free Press, 1979.

Impending Ethical Dilemmas in the Allocation of Health Care Services

IN THE PAST 20 YEARS, expenditures for medical care have increased very rapidly, blunting perception of the reality that health services are a finite resource relative to the potential demands of a community and the possibilities of biomedical science. The public highly values biomedical progress and supports investment of even greater proportions of our national product for medical care, but ultimately such expenditures must be balanced against other national priorities and personal needs.

The subsidy of medical care costs in America is generous, but even now the needs of the chronically ill, the uninsured, the poor and near-poor, and many other groups in the population are not addressed adequately. There are probably sufficient resources expended to provide a decent level of care to all, but our ways of organizing and financing care lead to significant disparities in availability of the range of services particularly essential for those with chronic handicapping disorders. American medicine has been impressive in providing to most the latest advances in the technology of acute care medicine; it has been less impressive in organizing and financing the sociomedical services required by those with more persistent and irreversible impairments.

It is ironic that a system of care so successful in preserving the life of a premature infant of just a few pounds, or that allows continued functioning of many patients through transplantation of organs or through maintenance on the artificial kidney, does so poorly in serving the chronic mental patient, or in assisting the frail elderly in retaining sufficient function to remain in their own homes. At the same time that we demonstrate our technological prowess in replacing the liver, experiment in the transplantation of mechanical hearts, or develop increasingly sophisticated ways of imaging the brain and other body organs with noninvasive technologies, we seem to find it increasingly difficult to house the homeless sick, to nurture the health of disadvantaged young children, and to prevent the incapacitated aged from becoming destitute before providing the medical and supportive assistance they require.

As a culture, we do far better in the application of a "technological fix" than in building complex social arrangements that must be sustained over time in coping with expensive, frustrating, and often intractible problems. This explains, in part, our willingness to invest hundreds of thousands of dollars to experiment with the transplantation of a single mechanical heart, but balk at relatively modest investments to reduce risk factors through programs of behavior change. The extension of a life in the flesh appears much more compelling than the prevention of "statistical deaths."

Underlying the discussions of science and technology, prevention and cure, and rehabilitation and efforts to support functioning are fundamental ethical issues relating to the role and responsibilities of the medical sector and its internal priorities. We think of ethical dilemmas and choices as focused at the individual level, but health policy formulation is in one sense an enterprise in applied ethics. Our views of health and illness themselves, the range of financing possible, the definition of what constitutes a medically relevant service, modes of payment, and the definition of providers eligible for payment—all implicitly involve many social choices and value judgements that shape the delivery of services and significantly impact the lives of patients and their families. Too often, what is defined solely as a financial or administrative judgment has enormous implications for who can be served, in what contexts, and within what range of alternative options.

Throughout this book I have argued that society, through its governmental processes, must make choices that establish the opportunities and set the constraints for how the health care system operates as a whole. The community should decide what proportion of its resources properly go to medical care as compared with other important needs, what priorities to give to researching and aggressively pursuing alternative disease and public health challenges, and the framework of equity that is to govern how the community's vast expenditures are to be allocated. It is through public dialogue, interest group activities, and the political and governmental process that these definitions become established and modified over time.

In supporting the merits of implicit rationing—that is, a system that establishes constraints but allows patients and professionals to work out accomodations that fit the variety of their needs, inclinations, and preferences—I have also suggested that the processes of administrative decision-making are too crude and rigid to accommodate adequately to the detailed complexities of sickness, the contingencies of people's lives, and the uncertainties of human transactions that span a community as culturally diverse as our own. They are also quite easily subjected to political pressures that erode the special character of medical services. While the society must set realistic limitations, every effort should be made to retain choices and options for patients and their doctors to do what best fits the contingencies of the specific situation.

Impatience with variabilities and inequities in practice encourage the search for explicit administrative rules that define the range of care to be made available in specific circumstances, specify when it is appropriate to use varying technologies, and the degree to which aggressive and expensive efforts to extend life should be made under varying circumstances. There are those who believe that these are important social choices that should be explored in public discussion, and that "society" should decide the difficult issues that advances in science and technology increasingly confront us with. The community should play a role through public discussion and its administrative agencies in deciding the relative emphasis on prevention, maintenance, and cure, the priorities for research and development, the overall strategy for insuring reasonable access to services for all citizens, and the balance of investment among children, the aged, and other dependents. But uncertain clinical circumstances that intimately involve the interest of patients and their families, are better resolved in private contexts among patients, their families, and physicians than by administators and regulators.

A viable concept of community depends on a certain flexibility of social arrangements, a willingness to allow varying groups to work out issues that affect them more than others without undue interference, and a certain inclination to "live and let live." The social system must set legal, ethical, and financial constraints, but when it needlessly legislates rigid prescriptions that impose a single worldview on people who differ in their life situations, values, preferences, and aspirations for the future it causes friction and divisiveness. Many matters, particularly those involving private concerns and deeply felt personal values and preferences, cannot be effectively prescribed. People with similar sociodemographic characteristics differ in their personal agendas, their preferences for care, their tolerance for pain and discomfort, indeed their desire to live when deathly ill. These are matters better left to health professionals and patients to negotiate than to public polling or bureaucratic mandates.

Professional discretion is never foolproof and mistakes and abuses certainly occur. But given proper protections the public good is better preserved by facilitating negotiation and communication between doctor and patient about the measures to be taken, than imposing these bureaucratically. Attempting to prescribe when people should be resuscitated, when heroic surgery should be attempted, when supreme efforts should be made to keep an irreversibly handicapped infant alive, and hundreds of similar decisions, cannot be formulated in a vacuum, without full knowledge of the complex contingencies.

Such discretion is not a license for physicians to impose their personal values in clinical situations. In many contexts a general consensus develops as to what range of behavior is reasonable, and physician peer review, ethics committees, living wills, and other instruments yet to be devised will serve usefully in helping develop a better-defined range of options and resolve difficult cases. The best ultimate protection for the patient, and our system of care, however, is to nurture trusting professional-patient relationships, and to facilitate resolving conflicts that arise from erosions of trust. The dilemmas of critical care and the impending possibilities of new life-extending technologies capture our imagination and justify our anxieties, but in the long run the integrity of the health care system will depend on appropriate processes of decision and resolving conflicts in a timely and constructive way.

A fundamental ethical responsibility of all health professionals is to respect the patient. The notion of respect is not an intangible symbolic notion; it refers to specific behaviors that are definable and measurable and includes freedom from coercion and informed consent. Patients have the right to receive accurate factual information about their condition and alternative options for care, including risks and benefits. They also have the right to refuse treatment or insist on options that are less radical than physicians may desire. Patients may want more or less information depending on personal tastes and predispositions, but patients typically want more information than they actually receive. Patients should, of course, be able to enter into agreements with physicians to delegate responsibility for their well-being and necessary choices. Respect also implies that, within the context of existing economic limitations and uncertainties about care, the medical decisions made should be solely on the basis of medical need and expected health benefits, and not on social, political, or religious criteria or on calculations of the "social value" of the individual patient. While some argue that scarce resources should be provided to "more valuable" persons, the intrusion of the issue of value is insidious and ultimately erodes the ethical foundations of medical activity as a neutral beneficent enterprise. In the real world of medical activity it is inevitable that such judgments intrude, but it would be folly to elevate them to principles of public policy. Finally, a system of care based on respect, but also with awareness of the inevitable inequality of power between the technical expert and the dependent patient, must have mechanisms to equalize power in instances of conflict.

Ethical Issues for the Clinician

My purpose here is more with exploring ethical issues inherent in the changing role of the physician from advocate to allocator, and thus my focus on macro issues, but there are compelling dilemmas at the clinical level that affect every clinician.[1] While it is easy to assert that medicine must respect the autonomy of patients to make their own life choices, it is not unusual for decisions to be necessary where patients lack competence to decide, communicate mixed messages about what they wish, or vary from one day to another about their desire to live or their wish to be resuscitated.[2] Perhaps the most challenging and difficult issue for many physicians is to learn to communicate openly and clearly with their patients, to discern their "true" intentions and desires in terminal or critical situations, and to listen and communicate deeply enough to appreciate the degree to which patients truly understand their situations and options and what their "real wishes" are. Even in ordinary interactions, much less in matters of life and death, surface assertions often hide far more complex feelings, ambivalence, and fears. However difficult,and it is difficult, physicians must learn to communicate clearly and honestly, but also with sensitivity, so that they do not destroy the optimism and hope that is vital to patients struggling with severe illness. This is more art than science, but it is a skill equal to high levels of technical competence.

In recent years, there have been many innovations both formal and informal that attempt to deal with the complicated decisions necessary when individuals lack consciousness or no longer remain competent to provide informed consent or make reasonable judgments. I trust that this is just the beginning of more comprehensive efforts to enhance the quality of decision-making consistent with our ideals of respect for persons under the illness contingencies that arise. While increasing numbers of such cases are coming to the courts, and the legal process must surely play a role in this complicated arena, medical care and medical decision-making cannot be solved constructively by shifting decisions from doctors to judges.

Under most circumstances sound decisions can be arrived at jointly among the health professionals involved, the patient, and family, but family members can have interests in conflict with the patient, be in disagreement among themselves, or be reluctant to make life or death decisions about loved ones. Living wills are typically drawn up by persons when well, giving instructions about their care in critical situations where they may not be competent to decide, but it is difficult for persons drawing up such documents to foresee future eventualities with the specificity that might be necessary at a critical time. Moreover, people who are well cannot easily imagine their situation or emotional ambivalence under circumstances where they are seriously incapacitated. For this and other reasons, the living will has been judged to be a less useful instrument for critical choices than many had hoped.

A more recent innovation, now embodied in law in Pennsylvania and California, provides for power of attorney for medical decisions,[3] not unlike that involved in commercial transactions, where the person legally designates another person who can make necessary decisions about their care should they become incompetent or in situations of terminal care. The California law is seen as more advanced in that it carefully specifies procedures and safeguards and prescribes the limits of action restraining the proxy decision-maker. Even when the patient lacks capacity, the designated decision-maker is expected to act consistent with the desires of the patient, and to the extent possible, the patient can state these wishes while competent in the power of attorney. If the situation is unclear, the proxy person is to act in the best interests of the patient and has the right of access to the patient's medical record and to be kept informed by the doctors providing care.

There is, of course, no adequate substitute for close communication between physicians responsible for decisions and critically ill patients and their families. This depends more on the development of trust and rapport and less on formal instruments such as living wills or power of attorney. Bedell and Delbanco[4] report that one out of every three patients who die at Beth Israel Hospital in Boston undergo cardiopulmonary resuscitation. They studied how 82 private physicians and 75 house officers planned for this eventuality involving 154 patients who received cardiopulmonary resuscitation following "sudden cessation of circulation or respiration, resulting in documented loss of consciousness." On the basis of questioning doctors, they found that about two-thirds had an opinion about their patients' attitudes, but rarely discussed it with patients even when they believed that patients should always participate in such decisions. In interviews with 24 competent patients who survived, they found that physicians' preconceptions about resuscitation were only weakly correlated with patients' actual preferences. No doubt, such communication is difficult and anxiety-provoking for the physician, and it's particularly difficult to discuss this sort of issue with patients not in immediate crisis who might become frightened by the discussion unless undertaken with great skill. There are no easy solutions, but this study, and experience more generally, points to the importance of developing physicians' communication skills and awareness in such areas of decision-making increasingly common in high-technology medicine.

Hospitals now more commonly have ethics committees to provide consultation on the management of profound ethical dilemmas inherent in the new technologies and possibilities of medical intervention. Neither ethics committees nor the other innovations discused are panaceas for the perplexing dilemmas that arise. But it is apparent that our efforts to think through, discuss, and test varying approaches provides a context for focused ethical consideration and the evolution of approaches that allow us to maintain respect for the person even in situations compromising the human qualities of personhood.

Ethical Dilemmas in Allocation

The President's Commission for the Study of Ethical Problems in Medicine and Biomedical and Behavioral Research grappled with the ethical implications of variations in the availability of health services. While they concluded that society has an "ethical obligation to insure equitable access to health care for all,"[5] they left large issues open by defining equitable access as being "able to secure an adequate level of care without excessive burden." There is a broad consensus in our society that people should receive necessary care; the debate truly becomes difficult in defining more clearly what "adequate care" is and what constitutes "an excessive burden." Concepts of adequacy change with advances in medical science and new technologies, and what we see as burdens is as much a matter of political philosophy as objective measures.[6] Social perceptions and politics will set the constraints and definitions of minimally adequate access; in the following discussion I focus on the organizational implications of rationing of medical care.

A variety of uncertainties affect access of services to the poor. As efforts are made to contain costs, eligibility criteria are more difficult to meet for Medicaid, and cost-sharing requirements have substantially increased in Medicare. The massive growth of profit-oriented institutions and services dilutes commitment to the poor and some 35 million uninsured persons, and the increasing shift of such patients to public hospitals puts great pressure on their ability to provide care comparable to that received by insured and more affluent patients. Moreover, as part of cost-saving strategies, Medicaid populations are increasingly locked into preferred provider organizations. The consequences of these trends create uncertainties that require vigilance.

Problems arise when demand for services is large and resources are limited. Services may not be available, and when they are, care is often rushed, relationships between health professionals and patients become impersonal, and communications, explanations, and opportunities for asking questions and obtaining feedback are limited. These problems affect minority-group patients or patients in lower socioeconomic circumstances more because they are more likely to be in programs that strictly ration care, while the affluent more frequently participate in programs characterized by open-ended budgeting or that have greater availability of personnel and other resources. Even when payment for care is available, as in Medicare or Medicaid, the poor are more likely to reside in areas with lesser concentration of facilities, making it more difficult for them to "cash in" on their entitlements.[7]

The disadvantaged and the poor may be penalized in rationed systems not because of discrimination but because better-educated clients are more adept at manipulating bureaucratic systems and more skillful in overcoming organizational barriers. They typically have higher expectations, are more aggressive, and learn to present their symptoms and needs in a way that achieves more rapid appointments and treatment. Nonfee types of rationing for some patients can be barriers as significant as co-insurance and deductibles and can have the same inequitable results.

In introducing new programs, there tends to be considerable exaggeration as to the benefits to be expected. Such rhetoric raises expectations that are not fulfilled. The marketing of new types of medical care plans, such as health maintenance organizations, is an example. When such plans are marketed, they usually promise a comprehenive benefit package, although there is often in reality a reluctance to provide some of the benefits advertised. Enrollment in an HMO is really an agreement between the enrollee and the plan to accept a situation of "constructive rationing," although such plans are not typically described to consumers in this way. For a lower premium, more comprehensive benefits, or both, the consumer implicitly agrees to accept the plan's judgment as to what services are necessary. The nature of this agreement is not usually made explicit, and these plans are often sold under a marketing rhetoric that distorts the situation.

In individual instances, deception and falsification are evident in some marketing efforts, but to dwell on these abuses misses the larger point. Even in the reputable plans, the scope of promised services is more than the plan hopes to provide, and a variety of barriers are put in the way of the consumer who attempts to obtain them. For example, enrollees are told that HMOs are organized to provide care as early as possible in sickness episodes. What they are not told is that HMOs eliminate economic barriers to access but replace these with a variety of bureaucratic impediments and limitations on the resources provided that keep enrollees from using too many services.[8] While HMOs may still be the "best deals in town"—and I am inclined to believe that they are—they are sometimes marketed in a way that is misleading to the consumer. Similarly, many of the nonprofit and for-profit insurance plans are so complex and described in such esoteric terms that even an expert consumer cannot easily evaluate them.

As the health sector becomes more commercialized overall, and health plans and hospitals compete for patients in an arena of greater cost constraints, we begin to see more efforts to dominate lucrative markets, to establish in the public mind a view that particular hospitals and chains offer exemplary technical services on the cutting edge of medical advance, and to avoid patients in need but who lack insurance. The orchestrated efforts of Humana to make highly visible and promote publicity for their efforts in mechanical heart transplantation conveys to the public the image that Humana hospitals offer the most advanced technology and technically proficient doctors. Although systematic data are difficult to obtain, there are increasing reports of emergency patients who cannot pay being turned away from for-profit and voluntary hospitals, and indications that whether the patient has insurance is taking precedence over critical need for immediate intervention.

The Health Care System and Tragic Choices

I have already suggested in prior chapters that given public support for medicine and advanced technology, it is highly unlikely that the American population would support the rationing of expensive high technology in the fashion characterizing England's National Health Service. While the public supports the elimination of waste and more stringent cost-controls on hospitals and physicians, such support is usually based on the belief that charges are too high, unnecessary procedures are too commonly carried out, and pointless heroic efforts are taken at the end of life often against the wishes of patients and their families. Few complain about enormous expenditures for chronic hemodialysis, perinatal intensive technology, coronary bypass surgery, or coronary intensive care because these are perceived, whatever their merits, as procedures that extend useful life, and the public is enthusiastic about government support for development of new lifesaving technologies. While it may be that the public has developed unrealistic expectations about what medicine can do at affordable costs, it is not likely to tolerate holding back on major technologies that offer hope for combating life-threatening diseases of significant visibility that they perceive can affect them and their loved ones.

Yet the emerging realities of technological advance suggest that we may soon be on the threshold of new technologies that can potentially assist large numbers of people but that are extraordinarily expensive and would, if made generally available, require vast expenditures. Some believe we have already arrived at this point. New immunosuppressive drugs make transplantation more viable than ever before, and we are on the threshold of major advances in transplantation of mechanical hearts and partial heart replacements. While experimental technologies are always more expensive than techniques once perfected, no one anticipates that transplantation of hearts and livers, for example, will be only trivial add-ons to already high medical care costs.

In short, we can anticipate situations where demand for new technology exceeds the community's willingness or capacity to provide for it. Many people presently die because of the shortage of human kidneys, livers, and hearts, yet we rebel at the idea that such organs should be sold to the highest bidder. We are not fully consistent on this point; while we support a voluntary blood donation system, there has been a long-established marketplace for buying blood from donors, particularly rare types. Some have seriously argued for a marketplace for kidneys, since individuals can sell one of their two functioning kidneys without serious dangers to life and health. The necessary personal match between seller and buyer in a "kidney marketplace" strikes us as more shocking than the impersonal sale of blood. But if a kidney middleman had the capacity, for a price, to indefinitely store bought kidneys in a more impersonal system that matched patient need against an available kidney bank supply, would we be less repelled?

It is in high technology areas where we face the stark reality of patient need against scarce resources in life and death situations that we see rationing with all its sharp edges exposed. These are indeed decisions that Calabresi[9] calls "tragic choices" in that they constitute situations in which there is no right decision. As he notes, any system we devise for choosing among lives has heavy external costs. In a pluralistic society in which differences exist in fundamental values, any explicit decision is likely to violate important concerns. The impossiblity of such choices, some have argued, should lead us to choose by lottery, or as Calabresi has suggested, possibly by alternating from one system of allocation to another.

The dilemma is not a new one—indeed, it has many similarities to past debates as to who should be drafted for the armed forces when the numbers needed are smaller than the eligible pool. All involuntary modes of selection and exclusion have large costs bringing to the forefront conflicts about the value of persons, inequities of class and race, and the manner in which special influence operates in a supposedly equitable society.

In the future we will increasingly face such tragic choices in medical care, and in all probability we will see many of the same preferential systems evolve that caused so much soul-searching in debates over the draft. While the idea of a lottery is inherently fair in adjudicating across value systems, it often impresses adherents of particular value systems as irrational and capricious, and it is not clear that the public would ever accept this as a mode of medical care allocation. There is, of course, the British concept of the queue, which effectively rations services in the highly underfinanced National Health Service. But even in Britain, the affluent commonly jump the queue through the private market. Such tendencies would be much greater in the United States where the population is more affluent and private markets and entrepreneurial interests more vital. It is difficult to conceive of the United States restricting the availability of any effective medical technology in the marketplace simply because government programs or even insurance companies will not pay for them. The extent to which public programs finance these technologies will depend on the inequities that result, the public awareness of these discrepancies, and the resulting tensions and political pressures.

Life is often unfair, and many inequities presently exist in allocation of medical care as in education, housing, and the administration of justice. We may lament the fact, but it seems likely that while the new technological advances may benefit us all, they will increase disparities in access and care among varying income groups. However strong the quest for equity, it is unlikely that we will restrict the entire population to levels of care characteristic of government supported programs however good the overall benefits. I suspect that medical care in the future will be organized more like higher education with the range of variation we see in public and private institutions, and a good deal of implicit rationing.

Mechanisms for Ethical Accountability

Throughout, I have argued that the community through public discussion and its political processes should set the financial constraints and framework of equitable access, but that implicit professional decision-making should decide the strategies of approach in individual cases. While the methodology for making tragic choices should be discussed in a broad value context, the dramatic instances, such as who receives a limited supply of hearts or livers, mask many smaller and less dramatic decisions that are pervasive in the allocation of medical resources just as they are in other areas. As the medical care process shifts toward greater concern with allocative decisions, we will have to devise new means of addressing difficult ethical issues and conflicts that develop between patients, professionals, and medical institutions. We will have to muddle through on many problems in devising responsive systems of redress. I conclude this chapter by considering some alternative possibilities. The integrity of the decision processes we develop may be as important as the actual allocative decisions in maintaining the respect and legitimacy of the medical care sector.

The current pattern of increasingly locking patients into specific systems of care limits patients' abilities to exercise alternatives when dissatisfied. Patients have more power and are less vulnerable to potential abuse when they have options. To the extent that medical care programs restrict choice, they are less likely to assist patients in representing their own interests. In theory, patients in the fee-for-service sector can exercise choice and, if dissatisfied with their medical care, can seek care elsewhere. Although location, geographic distribution of facilities and physicians, and other factors such as the patient's dependency may inhibit exercise of such choice, the patient, if sufficiently dissatisfied, can frequently go elsewhere. Both patients and physicians are aware of this, and in this sense the patient exercises a certain degree of client control.[10] Similarly, in the case of health-care plans, such as health maintenance organizations or different types of insurance programs, many consumers have a dual choice allowing them to exercise options if they are dissatisfied. Dual choice provisions have a double function not only in allowing a dissatisfied consumer to change plans but also in protecting the plans themselves from dissatisfied clients, who may create a variety of problems.

There are many instances—and these are frequently found in the public sector—in which patients have no effective choice. In many government programs, for example, patients who are dissatisfied with the care they receive have no market options because they cannot afford private care or because comparable facilities are not available. This lack of choice frequently applies to tertiary care facilities as well because such facilities are geographically more dispersed than other types of medical services. Thus, patients requiring specialized cancer care, or other more complex medical services, may also have few options as to the facilities they use.

Problems relating to lack of choice and potential abuse are more acute in public programs for the disadvantaged because this lack of choice is frequently associated with other factors that pose potential problems. Many programs for the disadvantaged, for example, depend on physicians and other health care personnel who are salaried and who do not depend on the patient's goodwill for their employment or remuneration. A variety of studies have suggested that in such circumstances client control is diluted, and patients frequently feel that physicians are less interested in them and less responsive to their needs.[8] Problems are further exacerbated by the characteristic imbalance between demand and resources, social distance and language barriers, and stigmatization and criticism of "welfare clients." Thus, programs of this type pose special, but not unique, problems of inequality of status, power, and dependence between patients and health care personnel.

The crux of the issue is the inequality between provider and patient and the extent to which these inequalities are growing with changes in the organization and provision of health care. Mechanisms are necessary, therefore, that contribute to narrowing these inequalities and that provide effective feedback to administrators and professionals as to the problems and experiences of patients. Possible mechanisms to close inequalities include effective grievance procedures and use of ombudsmen. A short description of each of these approaches follows.

Grievance Procedures

Increasingly, patients use medical institutions or are clients of programs for which there are no alternatives. Thus, if they feel their rights have been violated, they have little recourse but to complain directly to the providers, withdraw from using services, or initiate litigation. Patients are frequently reluctant to make direct complaints, and when they do there is no assurance of responsiveness. Similarly, withdrawal from service is not a serious option. Litigation requires considerable initiative and does little to resolve the initial problem when it occurs. Moreover, litigation is a highly formalized and time-consuming process that involves considerable costs for both the patient and the medical care system. Also, because the initiation of litigation is relatively infrequent and highly disruptive for all concerned, as in the case of malpractice suits, it results in a distorted pattern of compensation and poor resolution of existing problems.[11]

What is needed in any sizable program is a grievance procedure through which patients who feel wronged can make their problems and concerns known. Such a procedure would allow for relatively rapid mobilization to deal with problems early in their development, provide information to the institution concerning patients' dissatisfactions and concerns, and provide an opportunity to give feedback to patients who have unrealistic or misguided expectations. To be effective, such a grievance mechanism must be institutionally based and have *strong administrative support* to seek remedies to problems that are identified. Moreover, it must be structured so that it is *visible to patients*, so that *access* to patients *is high*, and so that the grievance process can be initiated without elaborate or formal preparation. For the most part, the mechanism would be used to achieve informal resolution of difficulties that arise in the patient care process, but under some conditions more formal procedures may be required. Such a grievance mechanism must include sufficient involvement of consumers or consumer representatives to insure that it does not simply deflect criticisms or problems. Moreover, procedures should be developed to allow staff to initiate grievances concerning failures and inadequacies of care in the program—staff are often familiar with problems and abuses but have no adequate way of communicating their concerns.

Most grievances can be handled informally with little cost. When a complaint is first made it should be recorded and some attempt made to resolve it quickly through consultation with the parties involved. When the grievance arises from real conflicts of interest or perspectives, and after an explanation the patient wishes to pursue the issue, more formalized procedures would exist for a hearing and an attempted resolution of the grievance. It is not difficult to specify the steps to follow in a grievance mechanism from rapid and informal resolutions to more formalized proceedings. The grievance mechanism could be adaptable to a wide variety of problems related to ethical concerns, and by its very existence might serve as a deterrent to at least some types of abuse. The existence of a visible grievance procedure provides some leverage for the patient in cases of abuses arising from the inequality of provider and patient. Through the maintenance of records of complaints it becomes possible to pinpoint troublesome areas of care and to inititate discussion as to the ways problems can be remedied. Also, the existence of a serious grievance process contributes to the consumer's sense of trust that the program is accountable.

The Ombudsman

As institutional medical programs become more complex, the opportunities for breakdowns in communication and coordination and for misunderstandings very much increase. Many of these problems can be corrected if there is someone available who understands the context and the types of problems that commonly develop and can communicate to the parties involved in the patient's care. Many hospitals in the United States have instituted ombudsmen programs, although they function more often to protect the institution's image and public relations than to delve very deeply into serious violations of patients' rights. In most such programs the ombudsman has limited influence to intervene when there are serious conflicts of interest, and the value of such persons is largely to improve communication. If we can assume the goodwill of most health care professionals—and I believe we can—then the ombudsman, despite the limitations inherent in the role, provides an opportunity to improve communication and to prevent the escalation of misunderstandings, and can assist patients in communicating their needs to health care professionals. Like the grievance procedure, the ombudsman program contributes to reducing the inequality in sophistication in understanding the medical setting between patient and health professional and provides an alternative to more inflexible rules and regulations. The ombudsman role can be established so as to increase advocacy for institutional change, and the ombudsman can be given the authority to initiate grievance procedures when informal resolutions of problems cannot be achieved.

Conclusion

The ethical problems in service delivery are both varied and complex, and there are real dangers in an approach that tries to respond to each new problem by writing new guidelines and rules. Such regulation in the aggregate not only involves high administrative costs but also feeds skepticism and contempt from those whose behavior the rules are intended to influence. More modest efforts, better fitted to the realities of organizational behavior, may induce a more sensitive response to the interests and needs of patients.

Inequalities in power between patients and providers are greatest and most troublesome when the patient lacks choice. Ironically, with growing competitiveness for patients among health care plans and physicians, affluent patients and those with good insurance may have greater countervailing influence. But the poor and uninsured, who face the largest inequalities to begin with, will face even more limited options with efforts to control cost in public programs. Employees who have health insurance as a fringe benefit are also increasingly being constrained in their choices because more employers are now motivated to limit their costs for health care benefits by locking employees into a single plan. In contrast, it is preferable for employers to offer the equivalent of a voucher, allowing the employee to choose among competing systems of care. However the insurance market evolves, problems will increase in a variety of situations where it is not feasible to offer more than a single site of care whether because of financial considerations, geography, or the complexity of sophisticated care necessary. It is far better to anticipate difficulties, and develop educational and other correctives, including more vigorous involvement of the health professions, than it is to revert to detailed regulation.

In the final instance, patients always have recourse to malpractice litigation, and increasing numbers of lawyers and doctors are active in this field. There are many strong opposing views on malpractice litigation, but it has some deterrence effect, and at times compensates injured patients. No one seriously maintains that the patterns of litigation and compensation that occur are equitable. Many influences have increased the significance of malpractice remedies: excessive patient expectations, depersonalized care, the dangers of complex and more risky technologies, and the greater willingness and ability to litigate.

The malpractice situation will not disappear, but we should do as little as possible to encourage its growth by developing alternative strategies that keep small conflicts from escalating into major confrontations. A constructive approach would be to encourage programs to develop adequate grievance mechanisms, ombudsmen, and other devices that facilitate communication and feedback relevant to troublesome problems. Medical care involves real conflicts of interest, but there are many areas where goodwill, effective feedback, and mutual respect would enhance the quality of services far more than either imposing new and complex external rules or encouraging greater resort to the legal process. In the final analysis, the most precious asset of medical activity is the trust that patients have had in doctors, nurses, and medical institutions. A prudent strategy would nurture and build on trust in every possible way. Its erosion would in the long run harm the true interests of both patients and health professionals.

References

1. Culver C, et al. Basic curricular goals in medical ethics. N Engl J Med. 1985; 312:253–256.

2. Burt R. Taking care of strangers: the rule of law in doctor-patient relations. New York: Free Press, 1979.

3. Steinbrook R, Lo B. Decision-making for incompetent patients by designated proxy: California's new law. N Engl J Med. 1984; 310:1598–1601.

4. Bedell S, Delbanco T. Choices about cardiopulmonary resuscitation in the hospital. N Engl J Med. 1984; 310:1089–1093.

5. President's Commission for the Study of Ethical Problems in Medicine and Biomedical and Behavioral Research. Securing access to health care, vol 1: report. Washington, D.C.: Government Printing Office, March 1983:4.

6. Engelhardt HT, Jr. Allocating scarce medical resources and the availability of organ transplantation: some moral presuppositions. N Engl J Med. 1984; 311:66–71.

7. Davis K. Equal treatment and unequal benefits: the Medicare program. Milbank Mem Fund Quar: Health Soc. 1975; 53(Fall):449–488.

8. Mechanic D. The growth of bureaucratic medicine: an inquiry into the dynamics of patient behavior and the organization of medical care. New York: Wiley-Interscience, 1976.

9. Calabresi G. Commentary on government decision-making and the preciousness of life. In: Institute of Medicine. Ethics of health care. Washington, D.C.: National Academy of Sciences, 1974:48–55.

10. Freidson E. Client control and medical practice. Amer J Soc. 1960; 65(January):374–382.

11. Mechanic D. Some social aspects of the medical malpractice dilemma. Duke Law J. 1975; January:1179–1196.

Epilogue

UTOPIAN HEALTH REFORMERS believed that if good medical care could be made available to the entire society, health could be enhanced to a point where expenditures for medical care would be much reduced. The architects of England's National Health Service, for example, assumed that once established, prevention and cure would reduce the incidence of disease and future costs.[1] The outcome, we know, has been very different, with large escalation of medical expenditures characteristic of all modern nations despite the widespread extension of medical care. Yet there are those who believe that we have the potential to achieve substantially a state of natural death, with people remaining in relatively good health until they reach the outer limits of a natural life span.[2]

In the past two decades the gains in longevity in the United States have been impressive, particularly among the elderly, and future improvements similarly are likely to be concentrated among the older segments of our population. While the elderly at any age are probably more healthy and have greater vitality than earlier cohorts at comparable ages, the increased numbers of old people, now commonly living into the eighth and ninth decades of life, will require

enormous expenditures of medical and social resources. Future progress in longevity is less likely to come from preventing infant deaths
or reducing deaths among adolescents and young adults related to
behavior and social development, than from delaying the occurrence
and progression of major chronic diseases during adulthood. Future
progress depends substantially on improved risk prevention that limits noxious behaviors among which smoking is the most damaging,
controls exposure to environmental risks contributing to accidents
and cancer, and facilitates screening and continued treatment of persons at high risk, such as those with elevated blood pressure.

But even when we successfully implement what we know, the successes of medical care create new vulnerable populations and new
needs. The low-birth-weight handicapped, who would have died just
a few years ago, will demand much medical care throughout their
lives. The elderly, however robust, will need more services simply
because they now survive for longer periods with serious chronic disease, disabilities, and limitations of function. Vulnerable persons,
because of the successes of medicine, now survive into adulthood,
marry and form families, thus transmitting genetic vulnerabilities to
their offspring, who constitute new populations of future need.
Modern medicine, as one commentator has put it, must adjust to the
"failures of success"[3] that confront us with new dilemmas and new
scientific challenges.

Health is itself a nebulous concept, redefined by each society and
generation in light of its values, the progress of medically relevant
science, the demands of the physical and social environment, and
new expectations and aspirations. As René Dubos so aptly put it:
" . . . health and happiness cannot be absolute and permanent values, however careful the social and medical planning. Biological success in all its manifestations is a measure of fitness, and fitness
requires never-ending efforts of adaptation to the total environment,
which is ever changing."[4]

I began this book by noting the extraordinary ferment in health
care organization reflecting the enormous escalation in cost in the
prior two decades, a new competitive spirit perhaps best exemplified
by the rapid growth of profit-oriented ventures, important advances
in biomedical science and technology, and the changing age composition of the American population. Throughout, a great variety
of policy issues have been noted and some explored in depth.

In concluding, I emphasize that the salient problems of the moment must not deflect us from a long-range view of the tough and persistent issues. In the final chapters, a variety of initiatives affecting the health and functioning of the elderly and the chronically mentally ill were examined. Building the infrastructures to implement these initiatives and to insure stability of organization and financing are matters to be worked on well into the future. Throughout we have repeatedly come back to the concept of the health maintenance organization, a new name representing forms of medical practice with many old roots in America and elsewhere. Efforts, as a matter of national policy, to elevate HMOs as a major care alternative is at least 15 years old, and while we currently place great importance on the growth of this minority sector it is yet to be a full-fledged competitor. Serious efforts to reform health care requires a long view, much persistence, and appreciation of the complex forces at work, often at cross-purposes.

Politicians typically take a short-term perspective, with one eye on the immediate pressing questions that have to be resolved and the other on the next election, which demands working within narrow limits. The best long-term policy may require unpopular short-term investments strongly resisted by the public and no prudent politician can be inattentive to such concerns. The central and most important dilemmas for policy are far-reaching and may require decades to resolve in any fundamental way. Thinking up new public policies and even legislating them are relatively easy matters in contrast to implementing desired programs so they achieve their intended goals.[5] While each year may bring some incremental changes, the long-term shape of effective social policy requires a clear long-term vision of goals and necessary successive changes, however incremental, that evolve in a consistent way toward achieving them.

Almost 25 years ago, Herman and Ann Somers, in a book on the organization and financing of medical care,[6] defined seven areas requiring from their point of view critical policy decisions. Much of the list, including such areas as controlling the rise of medical care costs, better organization of physician services, forging new patterns of public-private relationships, correcting the imbalance between hospitals and other facilities and rationalizing the system, and dealing with the cost and inappropriate use of drugs, are probably even more troubling today than they were then. In two of the critical areas—increasing the supply of physicians and increasing access of medical care—there is evidence of remarkable progress, but in each of these domains new critical problems also have emerged. We were remarkably successful in increasing the number of physicians trained, to the point that we now anticipate a substantial surplus. Also, while impressive progress was made in extending access of care to the poor and the elderly, the large numbers of uninsured still remains a problem not easily solved in the context of fiscal concerns and many poor persons are no longer eligible for Medicaid. Advancement is not necessarily linear and too frequently developments are retrogressive. The focus of concern and conditions change, public views may alter, and our solutions may themselves create unanticipated problems for the future.

The current context involves a curious mix of more forceful federal and state regulation with efforts to unleash the constraints on competition by encouraging competing health care delivery systems and more discriminating purchasers of medical care alternatives. On the private sector side, we see major companies taking a serious interest in the health care costs of their employees, at times self-insuring against medical care costs, but more commonly increasing deductibles, co-insurance, and introducing other incentives that encourage using less services.[7] Several major companies, such as Mobil, PepsiCo, and Xerox, have established flexible accounts for each employee to pay for varying out-of-pocket medical costs not covered by their basic insurance policy, such as co-insurance and deductibles. Employees who do not deplete these accounts are allowed to retain the unexpended balance as a bonus. The rationale behind such plans is that employees avoid unnecessary or marginally useful care to obtain the bonus, thus saving the basic insurance program, whose premiums are paid by the company, and themselves money.

On the public side, both the federal government and some states are showing muscle never before demonstrated. The introduction of DRGs under Medicare, and more recent proposals to "ratchet down" prices, as the new lingo goes, and extend similar price control systems to physicians and other providers reflects an attitude toward price regulation that is radical for health affairs. On the state side, tough negotiations between state Medicaid authorities with preferred provider organizations as in California, where the state successfully achieved large discounts through competitive bidding, suggests a model for large buyers of health services that will test the efficiencies of health services provision. Goldsmith has argued that:

> A major reallocation of the economic risk associated with health care cost is underway within the U.S. health care system. This reallocation spans public and private sector distinctions, and is, for the first time, significantly implicating patients and providers alike in society's health cost problem.[7]

Whether the system tilts more toward marketplace or regulatory solutions, or uses regulation to stimulate competition among health care plans and providers, is less important than our ability to maintain our long-term commitment to the value that access to medical care of adequate quality should be available in relation to need, and should not be rationed by age, income, race, region, or any other form of social discrimination. Constraints will surely continue and expand as new science and technology open unexplored but prohibitively expensive possibilities. While government cannot insure the entire population everything that biomedical science may make possible, it can insist on a basic minimum encompassing preventive needs, effective curative efforts, and the promotion of functioning and relief of unnecessary suffering.

The challenges inherent in these goals are not easy or inexpensive to implement, and the dynamic character of health-relevant sciences and the system itself calls for continuing reappraisals and readjustments. Despite our many problems, the United States has an impressive infrastructure of facilities and technologies, a large and exceedingly well-trained corp of health personnel, and an enormous per capita health care investment. These resources—organized rationally, balanced appropriately among varying needs, and directed intelligently, but without a heavy regulatory hand—offers impressive potentialities for the future.

In the final analysis, medicine, however efficacious, cannot substitute for the broader social and personal conditions that promote health. There is much in the world we can neither control nor predict, and often our fates are as much a product of change and luck as they are of our own intelligence and foresight. While individuals can do much to promote their own health and welfare, we understand only incompletely the links among knowing, willing, and behaving in accord with intention. The force of custom and culture, and the group incentives that energize routine social behavior, often affect our sense of belonging, meaning, and health more than conscious personal decisions. Healthful behavior, thus, must be encompassed within the common culture and everyday routines. Achieving this goes well beyond science or education. It involves fundamental issues on how we think about ourselves, our relations with others, and our ties and responsibilities to the social order and to the environment. There is no way of escaping Rudolf Virchow's essential insight that medicine is in essence a social science, and politics nothing more than medicine on a larger scale.[8]

References

1. Lindsey A. Social medicine in England and Wales. Chapel Hill: U of North Carolina Press, 1962:100.
2. Fries JF. Aging, natural death, and the compression of morbidity. N Engl J Med. 1980; 303:130–135.
3. Gruenberg E. The failure of success. Health Soc: Milbank Mem Fund Quar. 1977; 55:3–24.
4. Dubos R. Mirage of health: utopias, progress, and biological change. New York: Harper, 1959:25.
5. Bardach E. The implementation game: what happens after a bill becomes a law. Cambridge, Mass.: MIT Press, 1977.
6. Somers HM, Somers AR. Doctors, patients and health insurance. Washington, D.C.: The Brookings Institution, 1961, Ch. 25.
7. Goldsmith J. Death of a paradigm: the challenge of competition. Health Aff. 1984; 3:6–19.
8. Waitzkin H. The second sickness. New York: Free Press, 1983:71–75.

Index